## Praise for *Flourish*

"Every midwife should read this book. Everyone who loves or lives with a midwife should read this book. Perfect timing right now for our challenging midwifery world."
Anna Kent, author of *Frontline Midwife: My story of survival and keeping others safe*

"It's like a good dose of truth serum and a breath of fresh air."
Paula Cummins, Midwifery Educator, Black maternity experience activist

"It was like you were inside my brain and writing down all the feelings I can't express."
Maya, midwife

"I LOVE IT!!! It encapsulates the landscape so clearly and in a very accessible and articulate way. It has made me cry, and I say 'yes!' so many times as I read it. THANK YOU for writing this. I will put it at the centre of my reading list for students."
Dr Jenny Patterson, Midwifery Educator, Researcher into Midwife/Mother trauma

"There's nothing else out there like this book. Nowhere do we find all this in one place. It's raw, harrowing at times, but also like manna from heaven for midwifery leaders."
Edith Graham, NHS and healthcare leadership coach

"Filled with the truth as we know it, along with compassion, hope and practical ways for midwives to not just survive but flourish. Kate's wisdom and experience shine through, and will offer a reassuring hand to those who need it most."
Dr Jan Smith, CEO of Healthy You Ltd and author of *Nurturing Maternity Staff*

"What an impressive book – warm, encouraging and full of hope – essential reading for midwives at all stages of their careers! I have spent most of my academic career researching the emotional wellbeing of midwives. Often, I have felt at a loss when asked: 'So how can we improve things, both as individuals and as organisations?' Thank you, Kate, for showing us what an emotionally safe and supportive workplace could look like and how it could be possible for us to get there."
Billie Hunter CBE, Emerita Professor, Cardiff University

*See also last page*

T0124486

*For Robin, Madeleine and Ione*
*Your births – and your lives – inspire me always.*
*May you know the gift of purpose.*

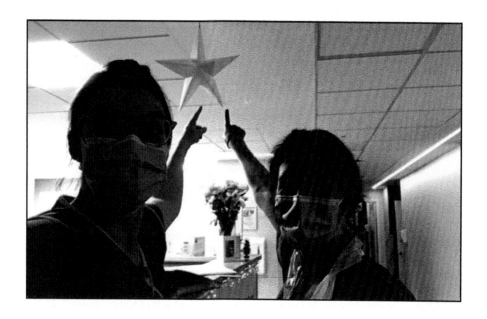

# FLOURISH

A practical and emotional guidebook
to thriving in midwifery

## KATE GREENSTOCK

*Flourish: A Practical and Emotional Guidebook to Thriving in Midwifery*

First published in the UK by Pinter & Martin Ltd 2023
reprinted 2023, 2024

Copyright © Kate Greenstock 2023

Illustrations © Jo Bradshaw 2023

All rights reserved

ISBN 978-1-78066-795-9

Also available as an ebook and audio book

The right of Kate Greenstock to be identified as the author of this work has been asserted by her in accordance with the Copyright, Designs and Patent Act of 1988

Index by Helen Bilton

British Library Cataloguing-in-Publication Data
A catalogue record for this book is available from the British Library

Printed in the UK by Ashford

This book has been printed on paper that is sourced and harvested from sustainable forests and is FSC accredited

Pinter & Martin Ltd
Unit 803 Omega Works
4 Roach Road
London E3 2PH

pinterandmartin.com

# CONTENTS

## Move the body

## Move the breath

## Move the mind

## Move the body

# FOREWORD

I've always been interested in the culture of healthcare organisations, especially maternity services, even before I knew what the term 'culture' meant. During more than 40 years working in the NHS as a nurse, midwife and then midwifery leader I have experienced first-hand how personal trauma can lead to transformation. Heart-breaking events including catastrophic outcomes, litigation, toxic leadership and bullying form part of my story, but I also had a successful and fulfilling career including exciting job opportunities, achievements and awards.

All this history defines me as a midwife as I continue in my quest to support and nurture others. While I can draw on my own experiences, I also need to expand my knowledge of the evidence available and learn from the experience and wisdom of others. How can I hear, engage, empathise and act to support student midwives and midwives if I don't have a bank of potential solutions to guide me and others towards a hopeful, positive future? I, like all midwifery leaders, must keep myself informed as I negotiate the ongoing issues in maternity services, where staff are reporting burnout, moral distress, and many are leaving or have already left.

Midwives are consistently engaged in emotion work as their position is to serve women and families during a transformational life event. The work becomes overwhelming and untenable when there is a lack of resources and support. If we are to transform maternity care and appropriately heal from the fallout of the Covid-19 pandemic and damning reports on maternity services then we must take action – and *Flourish* can help us.

The crisis we currently face provides an opportunity for change, to collectively improve and transform the culture of maternity care.

Positive relationships and human connection are protective for both providers and receivers of care. But individuals and teams need to know how this can be achieved, especially when the pressure is relentless.

This is where *Flourish: A practical and emotional guide to thriving in midwifery* is so valuable: it's a wonderful, joyous and much-needed support for midwives and midwifery leaders. We need to know how to stay psychologically and physically well both at work and at home, and Kate's open, warm approach shows us how we can thrive even in the toughest times, and how we can move forward despite the very real challenges we face.

The insights in *Flourish* are important for both individual practitioners and whole organisations, and the exercises in Part II encourage readers to reflect, explore, challenge and take action. Each sentence helped me to reflect on my own journey, not only as a practising midwife and midwifery leader, but as a mother and grandmother too.

*Flourish* can help us to deal with uncertainty and fear, embrace our vulnerability, examine our personal values and work on ourselves and with others to find a way forward. It is both compelling and easy to read, and I especially love the simple yet meaningful illustrations. The life-lessons and helpful insights apply to all areas of life, not just to midwifery. I hope you find that it supports your practice, and enables you to nurture others too.

Sheena Byrom OBE

# A LOVE LETTER TO
# MIDWIFERY LEADERS

*While we are all able to be leaders in our own lives and spheres of influence, this is a love letter specifically to those of you in positions of 'power' in the hierarchy.*

Dear midwifery leader,

It's hard from where you sit. You don't feel seen in the work that you do.

We see you right now.

It must be lonely sometimes, caught between the paralysis of not being able to tackle the biggest challenges, and the feverish action needed to keep the show on the road. No wonder you find it hard to talk to staff about what it really feels like to be a midwife in the current NHS. That's a scary place to go, especially when you want midwives to go on going on. And some midwives are angry, or very sad. Neither are easy to be with.

This book is for you too. It is not about setting up resistance to anything or anyone. Instead it is about taking the time to pose the most important question of all – is there another way? In acknowledging this, and walking through the experiences and exercises in the book, the purpose is to bring us together.

To sit with each other
Be with each other
Not fix it there and then
But share it…

This book invites a pause, which helps open up deeper conversations and a creaking door of hope. Your daily psychological challenges may look slightly different from the ones described in Part I, but whether you've lived the extremes of the peaks we're about to explore, you're still on the mountains where the air is thin. You too may experience 'unbearable feelings of helplessness in the face of service limitations'.[1]

So let us let this journey deepen our connection with colleagues, and learn together how we can deliver health – all round.

With compassion, and curiosity about what now and what next,

*Kate (on behalf of all of us)*

# INTRODUCTION

# HOW THIS BOOK WILL HELP

This book intends to support midwives to do two things: to name what's going on around us and within us, then to find and claim our distinctive place in the midwifery world.

You might be a newly qualified or early career midwife facing the challenges of finding your voice as well as your feet. Maybe you're an established midwife, and you feel like you have lost your way – and with it the impetus to readjust either yourself or the environment you work in. Perhaps you are a midwifery leader seeking to find the vocabulary to connect with your team, acknowledge what they might be feeling and reach out for resources and tools to support them (and you – you too) to thrive, learn and grow. This is about going beyond the old ways of survival.

As a guidebook, it is designed to take you on a journey – just like one you might pick up or scroll through on your travels. Think of it like a tour of discovery as we see more clearly how 'standard' maternity environments and practices might be impacting us personally, and then take an internal journey (which can be done with trusted colleagues if you choose) to reconnect with the core of our personality, purpose and passion. Prepare to experience the weight of your heavy heart. Then feel it lifting, shifting, opening once again.

*[Tuesday morning neighbourly conversation about midwifery]*
*'How wonderful. You must be loving it.'*
*[with nervous laughter and a tight smile, slightly cocked head]*
*'I'm doing it...'*

Designed to focus a wide-angle lens on the landscape we are working in, Part I will tackle the questions of status: what it means to be a midwife when society hails us as heroes, or with misty-eyed affection, yet our own regulatory body casts the shadow of potential villainy from the outset. It will ask what contradictions and self-sacrifice exist when working in a field regarded as a 'calling' or 'vocation'.

The Covid crisis has of course brought this question into relief. My favourite endorsement from the early pandemic was this one, inadvertently reminding us that while we would love to believe the 'celebrated heroes' narrative, we are more likely to feel like 'hore's' (sic), offering services to strangers for cash with little time for the human-focused patience and kindness these intimate acts require.

This guidebook will explore the contradictions of the notion of individual resilience, a word too often used as a metaphorical stick and treated like a character trait or competency to be weighed and

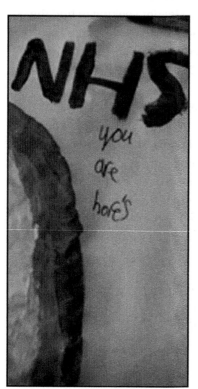

measured in the individual midwife, separating her/him from context and the significant organisational and systemic sources of stress.

The landscape will take us to explore places barely mentioned in midwifery training or practice: to the bubbling, semi-silent volcano of trauma experienced by midwives. It will lead us to question the impact of trauma on a midwife's experience of her own pregnancy and birth and her subsequent practice. It will guide us to the valley of moral injury as we live and work in ways that undercut our deeply-held values. It will take us to the hazardous, oxygen-starved heights of inevitable compassion fatigue, where the brain gets confused and thinks the only answer is to press on regardless, working more rather than less, just to survive. We will see how the thirsty desert lands of burnout make us more vulnerable to both trauma exposure and compassion fatigue. We will examine the cultures of leadership we swim through day by day; the historic legacy of what is tolerated and role-modelled. We will see how vulnerability can beat armour in shaping alternative, courageous environments.

And we will find our way back 'home'.

And by this I don't mean a boring or prosaic place. I mean a place where the fire of our original BIG WHY – our sense of motivation for being a midwife – crackles once again into flame in the hearth; where we reconnect to our values, strengths, the world we want to live in and our unique voice; where we find and claim our tribe of truly like-minded buddies or role models who inspire and encourage us. This is where the array of exercises in Part II will support you to a place of discovery – of coming home to YOU. From this place of warmth and conviction you are no longer stuck with the old stories or postures, with the disheartened shoulder shrug, but can make real, rich and raw choices as to what's next from a place of clarity about who you really are and what you most want.

## MIDWIVES MATTER

There are so many reasons to write this book. The research is clear and the reality is played out daily with colleagues signed off with stress and overwhelm, or living with depleted energy, drained vision and a sense of loss of purpose and expectation. We know from the 2019 Work, Health and Emotional Lives of Midwives (UK WHELM) study commissioned by the Royal College of Midwives[1] that 83% of midwives report moderate and above levels of burnout on a validated scale. 66.6% of the 2,000 participants stated they had thought about leaving the profession within the last six months. We also know from the application of the same data to early career midwives in a pre-Covid 2020 study[2] that early career midwives are disproportionately affected by the pressure of these environments. Options to take control of workload are limited or non-existent on a reactive labour ward or subject to a packed clinic 'list', leading to a feeling of helplessness or paralysis – a 'stuckness' which can add to the emotional toll. Continuity of carer models can offer a more positive alternative, but we are currently in a turbulent phase of re-experimentation with these ways of working.

The Covid-19 pandemic has added unexpected pressures and fears into a challenged system already suffering from little slow time, few intact teams, sparse attempts at reflection and a disconnect from some well-meaning human resource initiatives aimed at wellbeing, which often require midwives to access them in their own time. Indeed a 2021 RCM survey of 1,581 midwives showed 57% planning to leave the NHS in the next year.[3] Nearly half of midwives who choose to stay in the profession choose part-time work, in spite of the inevitable financial impact, as a way of asserting some control and balance in their lives.[4] Sally Pezaro's 2021 work shows one-third of midwives persistently misusing alcohol and other drugs to cope with stress, with 10% of her self-selected sample of 623 admitting to coming to work under the influence of alcohol and 6% having taken other drugs.[5] The rapid coalescence of the 33,000 strong March with Midwives movement in late 2021, in the midst of a growing staffing crisis, has highlighted in the media personal narratives of trauma, bullying and self-harm,[6] alongside systemic issues of toxic work cultures and chronic short-staffing.[7] Black, Brown and Mixed Ethnicity midwives suffer multi-layered disadvantages and direct discrimination:[8] they experience the psychological and physiological 'weathering' effect of ongoing macro and micro-agressions,[9] and are disproportionately involved in disciplinary proceedings, with disproportionately worse outcomes.[10]

I recall the end of a long shift in a grubby changing room strewn with scrubs; midwives all around me half joking about taking a supermarket job stacking shelves for comparable rates of pay, better conditions and a nicer uniform – and it half breaking my heart. That highly trained, intuitive, compassionate midwives would walk away is devastating enough. The hardened, unbroken part of my heart which understands completely is perhaps even more worrying.

Visionary midlife midwife Amity Reed's 2020 description of her career reads like a body blow. She details her retreat from enthusiastic gatherer of volunteers and resources to refurbish areas for staff and families, to thwarted, defeated midwife, receiving neither encouragement nor even a response from those with the power in the hierarchy to 'authorise' this mini project. Amity empathises with those very leaders who have just too much crossing their desk to focus on key opportunities to empower their people, *and* goes on to describe it as one of the significant events in the steady decline of her mental health.[11] It certainly demonstrates the antithesis of the culture of ABC (Autonomy, Belonging and Contribution) espoused by the recent King's Fund review of how to support nurses and midwives to deliver high quality, compassionate care.[12]

Of course this is not the experience of all. #JFDI (Just Fucking Do It) badges sported by obstetricians and midwives in another London trust are a light-hearted assertion of autonomy and spontaneous team work over NHS bureaucracy. Having run a marathon to raise funds to pay for beautiful friezes for the walls of labour ward rooms, teams came in on days off to work together to do the decoration. We know from the research that proactive behaviour among midwives is a protective factor against burnout.[13] ABC was very much in evidence: individuals collectively seizing the day and bringing the whole of themselves to work – their passions, values and what they know works for families. They were able, in that moment, to reunite role with soul.[14]

## WHO AM I TO HELP YOU REUNITE ROLE WITH SOUL?

As both a practising midwife and an experienced life and career coach, I have a distinctive perspective. I have found joy in my 15 years of coaching work reconnecting people to their values and sense of self, enabling them to see themselves as creative, resourceful and pioneering in their chosen domain. Given that who we are (in any given moment) is how we choose to work, this book is an opportunity for role to meet soul and take a stroll together; for that conversation to be a collective sigh of relief and discovery which then creates action and momentum. I am also a story-teller. I understand the learning power of hearing others' stories, and as midwives we deal in stories like precious currency. I have therefore included stories in the book – of midwives and obstetric colleagues who have developed their thinking about flourishing against the odds, often after personal suffering.

And it's not all about the individual midwife. Our more recent and understandable hyper-focus on stress-busting and self-care misses the interconnectedness of the self, the system *and* the organisation. I will hold this integrated perspective throughout.

## HOW TO USE THIS GUIDEBOOK

I intend for us as midwives to use this book either individually, in trusted pairs or in small groups, to enable us to rediscover our mojo, to stay in midwifery in a way that works, or to actively choose to leave – in order to thrive as individuals. First read through Part I and work through the accompanying reflective questions if you choose. You can expect to find these questions at the end of each chapter. Sometimes the journey through the psychological realities of midwifery might feel intense, especially if it closely mirrors your own experience. Know that if you feel overwhelmed on the oxygen-starved heights of the 'mega mountains', that even in Part I there is respite and hope: text boxes ask 'What if…?', inviting us to take a deep breath from the oxygen canister and reimagine how we might take small, powerful steps to work and communicate differently. The Part II exercises will bring a feeling of stable ground and a sense of clarity about who you

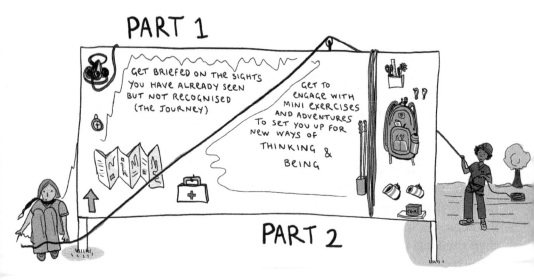

PART 1

GET BRIEFED ON THE SIGHTS YOU HAVE ALREADY SEEN BUT NOT RECOGNISED (THE JOURNEY)

GET TO ENGAGE WITH MINI EXERCISES AND ADVENTURES TO SET YOU UP FOR NEW WAYS OF THINKING & BEING

PART 2

are and your purpose as a midwife. They will also give you a backpack full of strategies, tools, mindsets and resets, first for survival in the moment and then choosing flourishing. You can do the exercises alone, with your chosen accountability partner or a small group of trusted colleagues. The most exciting thing about this work of discovery is that it will serve you throughout your career and in every corner of your life. Grieve, Breathe, Step Back and Reimagine...

Just to add, if Part I doesn't feel like it reflects *your* experience of life in midwifery, stay with the journey anyway: there is lots for you here. Ask yourself, how might I gently look at events over the course of my time as a midwife and see where I have chosen to numb rather than feel, to distance from myself or others? Ask how reading this book might deepen your connection with colleagues.

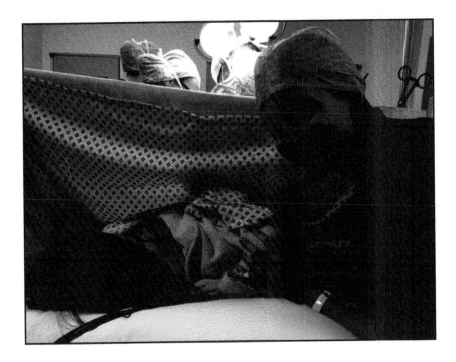

# PART I

# THE EMOTIONAL LANDSCAPE OF MIDWIFERY

# CHAPTER I

# HERO OR VILLAIN: THE PROBLEM OF THE STATUS OF MIDWIFE IN THE NHS AND IN POPULAR CULTURE

Never has it been more obvious to midwives that there is a mismatch between our idealised status in society and the feeling on the ground. It is rare that I speak to a woman over 35 who *doesn't* say 'I would have loved to be a midwife', or at the very least 'I can't even imagine how wonderful that must be'. With men it's often a conversation-stopper, which in itself is a mark of silent respect. Adverts, especially at Christmas, by major disposable nappy brands reinforce the image of the valiant twinkly-lighted heroes of the day and night, doing the 'best job in the world'.

There is a reason why the BBC series *Call the Midwife* is commissioned to film its fifteenth series by 2026: it makes us feel good. I know midwives who watch it to soothe themselves after a difficult day on the wards. For a whole hour, our fundamental contradictions are named or resolved, and kindness rules. The flow of tears allows adrenaline to leave the system.

In global midwifery terms, we are also pointed to 'Our Frontline Heroes'.[1] An additional 900,000 trained midwives, representing an increase of one-third, 'can save 4.3 million women and babies each year'.[2] There is no doubt that trained midwives save and enhance lives across the globe. But the overwhelming scale of figures like these, as well as headlines about 'heroes', raise the stakes for superhero midwives trying to navigate their working lives.

New parents bolster this culturally idealised view of midwifery, addressing the midwife on shift for their labour and birth with oxytocin-soaked words of appreciation and night shift-ready sugary gifts. As midwives we will often reinforce this image on social media, sometimes understandably seeking to communicate a little of what we do by celebrating or mourning an event, a connection or a gift with a phrase like 'makes it all worthwhile'. Parents' own 'couldn't have done it without you' statements of thanks meanwhile are unquestionably kind, largely untrue, and I would argue can increase the sense of disconnection/dissonance with what a midwife is often feeling about her role – and herself. Listen to the echoes of shame and guilt in these reflection statements from newly-qualified midwives about the reality of a shift:

> 'Honestly, I really didn't or couldn't do the very best for that woman/family.'
> 'I didn't speak up for her when it mattered most.'
> 'I went with the flow of the system and what was expected... it's just easier I guess.'[3]

Set this ambivalence against Apache pilot (and midwife's husband) Steve Osterholzer's description of midwifery:

> 'Being a midwife is similar to being an Apache pilot. That may sound strange, but it's true. One may suppose flying gunships in combat is as far removed from delivering babies as can possibly be, but the truth is, there are strong parallels. Both require remaining calm under immense pressure. Both require many years of demanding education. Both require courage and great technical skill. Both require making decisions which can literally mean life or death: where, if you make a mistake, a human being – be it a man alive for 60 years or a baby girl alive for 60 seconds – can die in your hands.
> Midwifery is a calling.
> Midwifery is a life dedicated to the service of others.
> Midwives are heroes.'[4]

## THE TROUBLE WITH HERO STATUS

The truth is we're confused. We want someone to acknowledge the drama and the courage, the distinct place of midwifery, as Sheila Kitzinger described it, 'on the threshold of life, where intense human emotions – fear, hope, longing, triumph and incredible physical power – enable a new human being to emerge.'

She goes on:

> 'Her vocation is unique. The art of the midwife is in understanding the relationship between psychological and physiological processes in childbirth. Rather than being the provider of a technical service to support a doctor, or someone who scuttles around getting ready for an obstetrician and clearing away after him, her skills lie at the point at which the emotional and biological touch and interact. She is not a manager of labour and delivery. Rather, she is the opener of doors, the one who releases, the nurturer. She is the strong anchor when there is fear and pain; the skilled friend who is in tune with the rhythms of birth, the mountain tops and chasms, the striving and the triumph.'[5]

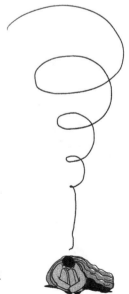

Yes, we went into midwifery, most likely with a sense of purpose, maybe even a sense of vocation. The word vocation comes from the Latin *vocare* 'to call' or be called. And this is the tricky bit: it presupposes self-sacrifice on the altar of calling. Even the Cambridge dictionary describes vocation as 'a type of work that you feel you are suited to doing and *to which you should give all your time and energy*' (my italics).[6] That all sounds really worthy, or worthwhile at least? Our role models or leaders are modelling going without breaks, staying beyond the 12.5 contracted daily hours, or doing 'just another bank shift'. Isn't that what *you* would do in service of a vocation or the women and families you serve?

Except that we feel like we are dying inside. And as we will discover in the next chapter, without proper rest our cognitive functioning is impaired, empathic strain leads to irritability with families and systems, cynicism and increased moral distress. It's a spiral.

Understandable attempts have been made to discourage the use of the phrase 'a calling' to describe the role of the modern university degree-qualified midwife with her or his enquiring scientific mind and justified request for decent pay. Yet the reality is this: it's not just a job. If it was, we wouldn't do it. It's too tough. Being a midwife has become mixed up with our identity. Participants in Bloxsome, Bayes and Ireson's 2019 in-depth study of 14 Australian midwives said that being a midwife represented who they were as a person: 'it's who I am… it can't be undone'.[7] Many of them used the phrase 'calling', adding for example that they would do it for free if they could. The UK WHELM 2019 study of 2,000 UK midwives found (paradoxically, perhaps, alongside extremely high levels of stress and burnout) midwives taking pleasure in their work and experiencing their identities as midwives as a source of pride and self-esteem.[8]

Samantha Batt-Rawden, a senior UK-based registrar in intensive care medicine, describes in *The Independent* newspaper in May 2021 the detrimental impact of the self-adopted or superimposed superhuman status of health professionals, even before the Covid pandemic. It leaves, she says, no room for the hero to be human, and to be asked 'how are you?'. The hero image has been further co-opted, she feels, 'to justify increasingly unsustainable working conditions in the NHS, without care for the needs of those who care for others.'[9]

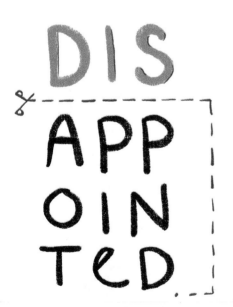

A binary narrative appears, especially in the media, of angels and heroes on the frontline, and of burned-out staff, in danger of succumbing to post-traumatic stress disorder. Both ends of the narrative depersonalise the health professional and leave less space for the conversation and cultural change needed for healthcare workers to live within a normal ebb and flow of human life including illness and health, both physical and emotional.[10]

For midwives, idealised status doesn't leave the space to name the emotionally profoundly demanding nature of the work.[11] And why is that important? Because if we can't name it, we can't easily see it. We are swimming in our own murky waters, shrugging our increasingly passive shoulders, saying that 'it's just the way it is', with a serious lack of interventions supported by evidence that could offer support to midwives and student midwives experiencing psychological distress at work.[12] Psychologist and maternity ally Jan Smith's 2021 book *Nurturing Maternity Staff* repeatedly addresses the psychological need for acknowledging the emotionally challenging environment, and for training students to be able to see it and actively choose to work in maternity departments making efforts towards psychological safety.[13] More on this in Chapter 9.

## THE FEAR OF BEING THE VILLAIN

There is a dark underside to the hero narrative. It goes like this: you can be a hero until you are the villain.

> *'I am tired and worn out and am concerned that if this continues, I might make a tragic mistake.'* Midwife[14]

Of the clinical negligence claims notified to us in 2021/22, obstetrics claims represented 12 per cent of clinical claims by number, but accounted for 62 per cent of the total value of new claims; almost £6 billion.[15]

Every midwife has a vague notion of this in the back of her mind. There is a doom-laced playlist playing, full of stories on rotation, which is mainly indistinct, but with sudden sharp interjections of the actual faces and names of families for whom something has gone wrong, or of colleagues who are under investigation. The fear of 'investigation' is strong. As one early career midwife put it, 'It is terrifying sometimes the pressure we have, the fear of litigation, the fear of something awful happening.'[16]

**What if** we were to build a system where any staff induction or welcome included the following messages to set some of the foundations for psychological safety?

- You do something hard.
- Which puts you at risk of psychological harm.
- It also puts you at risk of physical harm (think bad backs and type 2 diabetes from night shifts – see p.p. 64-65).
- Your chosen work also introduces an aspect of vulnerability and unpredictability into your life as things can and will go wrong at times.
- We acknowledge that and are here to support you.
- Here are YOUR agile learning team (new name for 'risk' team?) who know that incidents are usually complicated and involve many people and circumstances.
- When (not if) you are involved in the aftermath of an event, our first priority will be to look after your psychological safety. We know that blame is painful and isolating to individuals, does not reflect the nuance of the case and hampers all attempts to learn collectively and go on doing our jobs.
- That's why we make you our priority, while we also take care of the family involved.
- We also know that you (all colleagues) respect the story of an event as unknown. We understand that discussing an incident is often a response to your own fear of it being 'you next' or out of compassion for your colleague. We know from the research that half-storytelling fuels fear rather than reduces it and increases the likelihood of secondary traumatic stress in midwives.[17] It is more likely to make your colleague feel isolated and vulnerable. We encourage you to guard your heart and theirs.
- We are here to support you.

No midwife would object to a sense of rigorous accountability in a profession where lives and wellbeing are at stake, but the chasing down of that very accountability can often sacrifice the lives and wellbeing of midwives themselves. It can create this cycle:

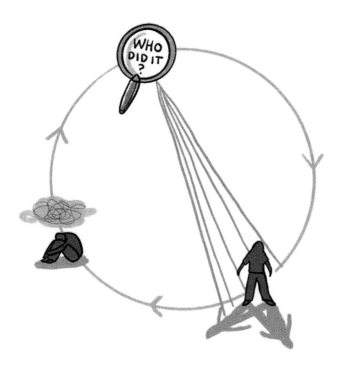

## WELLDOING 3, WELLBEING 0

Rachel Morris, a GP and coach who hosts the excellent 'You Are Not a Frog' podcast, calls well-meaning wellbeing offerings the 'fruit and bicycles approach'. As if a basket of fruit (occasionally seen in practice during Covid peaks) and a cycle to work scheme can affect the baseline of employee 'well'ness.[18] While dismissing such initiatives may be a little harsh, it is true that even where hospital or trust wellbeing services are offering potentially helpful solutions (including talking therapies/listening services – invariably accessed in your own time), we know that a lunchtime yoga session is certainly not accessible to a midwife who has no control over when in the day her break will be. Trust/hospital wellbeing services can feel very separate from the actual work, the location, the feel of what is happening on the ground.

What trained support there is in maternity, such as in the person or persons of the PMA* team doing their very best to be the source of tea and comfort for midwives away from the 'scene', can still feel distant and inaccessible because of the pervasive sense of:

> *'I just can't stop because if I do… then*
> - *my colleagues will suffer even more*
> - *I will somehow be marked as 'not tough enough'*
> - *something will get missed*
> - *I will have a tortuous end to my 12.5 hour shift trying to make up for time spent trying to recover my equilibrium.'*

What is needed is more training for leaders on the ground to recognise signs, articulate them with compassion and offer practical help and psychological first aid which centres on remaining in connection with that person. More on this in Chapter 8.

---

\* Professional Midwifery Advocate: a midwife or midwife team trained to advocate for midwives and listen to midwives and families, in England.

# CHAPTER 2

# OCCUPATIONAL HAZARDS

*'I suffer from a condition called being human.'* [1]
*This might make it difficult for me to work at my very best in this*
*environment. What reasonable adjustments might be possible?*

The first thing you do when you go on a journey is to find a map,
unfold it, or pinch the screen to get a sense of the lie of the land, the
characteristics of the landscape, the mountain ranges to cross or
obstacles to navigate. We're going to picture the following big five
mountains of maternity work. It's possible that you've never seen
them mapped out before, but you know what it feels like when you
slam into one of them.

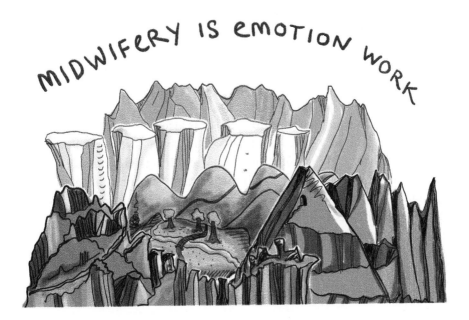

## MIDWIVES – LEADERS – EDUCATORS: THIS IS FOR EACH OF US

The aim of this section is to give language to the events and emotions we as midwives experience, whether persistently or occasionally. It is to give language to midwives as individuals, affirming the experience. It is also designed to give language to midwifery leaders to increase our capacity to acknowledge the very real daily challenges to our own and our team's emotional health. That acknowledgement alone can create a new measure of 'safety'[2] and encourage pioneering and courageous conversations about caring for each other within the profession.

It is also intended to focus us on a hope and a future: the major changes achievable by taking small steps at a university and newly qualified level. I remember my mixed feelings in response to a revelation in my final student year from our exceptionally emotionally controlled lecturer who, in her days as a clinical midwife, had been so angry about substandard care that as she left her then workplace in floods of tears, she kicked her own car and sobbed all the way home. I felt affirmed in that moment that it is indeed that hard; and that overwhelming emotion is a normal human response. And yet I was disappointed that it had taken until the third and final year to hear of the broken moments. It was as if our educators perceived that we somehow hadn't been ready; that we needed to be trained to the system ('it's how it is; do it or die') before we were 'resilient' enough to touch their red-hot emotional fallout, even though we were being burned by the equivalent every day in placement, yet not quite able to name what was happening.

So the language offered in this section is also here to challenge and encourage midwifery educators to place the psychological challenges of the role front and centre in the course, requiring vulnerability from leaders and teachers. What if that were to help 'normalise' the inherent anxieties and contradictions in being a midwife while providing students with a usable psychological language and understanding to enable reflection, which could in turn encourage safety, resilience and self-care?[3]

This is exactly what Lucie Warren, Billie Hunter and team are attempting with the midwifery programme students at Cardiff

University: enabling an early grasp of the language describing the psychological challenges and symptoms the students will face. They have a thread woven throughout their BMid degree courses supporting students to reflect on themselves, their experiences in practice and how to actively use the resilience repertoire[4] developed in their 2014 research with self-identified 'resilient' midwives.[5] They are keen for their students to develop the emotional language, capacity and courage to actually live out the NMC standards of proficiency 2019:

> *5.14 ...how to recognise signs of vulnerability in themselves or their colleagues and the actions required to minimise risks to health or well-being of self and others*
> *5.15 ...awareness of the need to manage the personal and emotional challenges of work and workload, uncertainty, and change; and incorporate compassionate self-care into their personal and professional life.*[6]

The students are encouraged to use the Three Good Things exercise for reflection, developed by Martin Seligman, the 'father' of positive psychology. This, alongside the repertoire, has been embedded into the All Wales Midwifery Practice Assessment Document. The exercise helps learn new pathways to shed negative biases in seeing and remembering events, and prompts students to notice the positive, and practice carving the brain pathways of gratitude, a vital life skill and an absolute lifeline in hard-pressed environments. When returning to university after time in practice, lecturers encourage and challenge the students using the ABC model,[7] now a core element of cognitive behavioural therapy (CBT) work, enabling students to slow down and explore how Activating events (A) have triggered Beliefs (B) (which may or may not be true). Those beliefs (not the event itself) have created Consequences (C), feelings, self-judgements, behaviours and so on. Cardiff students get to train their brains from the outset in not believing their own thoughts and seeing the new learning, story or possibility! See Part II, p187 for an easy to use extension of the ABC model if you want to try it out yourself.

So amid the mega mountains of midwifery, and the looming

shadows they cast, there is positive work happening. The RePair project on reducing attrition rates[8] is creating projects focused on stronger transitions into the newly qualified experience. A new injection of government funding in March 2022[9] is specifically meant to target sustaining midwives in practice, particularly in the early years. Extra funding is also enabling a start to be made in training UK Professional Midwifery Advocates in midwife-focused trauma-informed practice.

And yet, as Warren and Hunter cautioned back in their 2014 research on midwifery resilience, and as re-emphasised in the final Ockenden report in 2022, 'Workplace challenges, and how these may be approached in ways that are resilient and sustainable, need frank discussion rather than glossing over.'[10]

Let's go first to the air we breathe.

# CHAPTER 3

# MIDWIFERY AS EMOTION WORK

The mountains on our map overlap and intersect. Those who traverse the mountains may experience some of the same symptoms and see the same views. And the air they breathe is the emotion work of midwifery. This may sound obvious. But midwives report that it is often *this* crucial aspect of midwifery which feels under-appreciated or unacknowledged.[1] How many of these daily dilemmas have you acknowledged as involving emotion work?

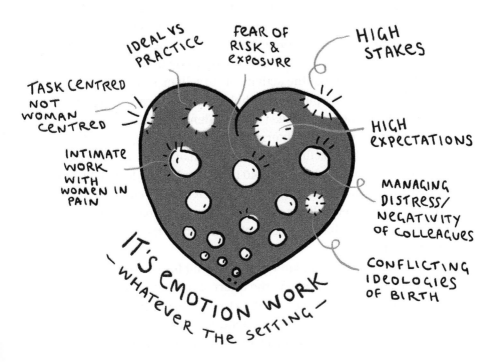

Borrelli, Spiby and Walsh's 2016 work on first-time mothers'
perspectives of a good birth midwife illuminates just how complex
and intense this emotion work can be in an intrapartum context. The
researchers assemble the 'kaleidoscopic midwife' from their findings,
used to describe:

> 'a midwife who is "multi-coloured" and ever changing in the light of
> the woman's individual needs, expectations and labour journey, in
> order to create an environment that enables her to move forward
> despite the uncertainty and the expectations-experiences gap...
> harmonising relationship-mediated being; knowledgeable doing;
> physical presence; immediately available presence.'[2]

It's exhausting just to write or read about the many layers of emotion
work present in this moment, let alone to do it!

## EVERYDAY CONTRADICTIONS REQUIRE EMOTION WORK

Daily intensive emotion work is also needed in managing the
dissonance in many settings between the way a midwife may want
to be 'with woman' and the organisational practices which she sees
as potentially harmful. There is the ongoing emotion work in living
with the knowledge that the activity of surveillance (such as CTG use)
required to seek out a possible pathology might be causing a deviation
from normal in the first place.[3,4] On an antenatal ward, a midwife
might experience a (brief) internal battle introducing potentially
unnecessary risk by facilitating an induction of labour at 40 weeks
for a healthy woman who turned 40 in July and is due to give birth in
August, or a woman with gestational diabetes that is consistently well
controlled with diet. Policies and pathways may be based on evidence
which may be less than robust, or place a woman the wrong side of a
generalised 'line'.

The midwife may hear later of the difficult birth stemming from
this induction process and feel the internal conflict of not having
challenged its original premise. She also knows in her heart of hearts
that resisting the 'institutional momentum'[5] involves strong emotional
energy, which she currently can't afford to expend given the five other

couples arriving for induction this morning. Her heavy heart also tells her that given the fear-based conversations that this woman is likely to have had in advance about the risks to her baby from her 'faulty' body, she will be primed to be taken in by the 'symbolism of safety: the promise that medical settings and procedures are always safer for birth than non-institutional settings and physiology-supporting practices.'[6] She sighs to herself and facilitates rhetorical autonomy – meaning she 'consents' the mother for induction while fully acknowledging only to herself the inadequacy of the process. All this internal frustration, questioning and sadness is emotion work. It takes its toll. Interestingly, Billie Hunter identifies these inherent conflicts as being strongest in newly qualified, student and continuity of carer midwives who tend to advocate strongly to be 'with woman'.[7]

> *'Above everything, not giving women and babies the care they deserve is the worst aspect.'* Early career midwife[8]

There is emotion work in managing 'risk' and its sister 'fear': what Mandy Scamell calls 'the latent worries that lurk in the back of the midwife's mind and drive her practice',[9] causing what she hopes are invisible 'little feet flapping about like mad' under a swan-like composure.[10] An early career midwife described this work of 'shielding' families as a source of satisfaction: 'knowing that I have made a difference to a family whilst they remain unaware of the strain I am under through excessive workloads and poor staffing'.[11] When we become aware of the reality that families actually *feel* the tension between soothing midwifery talk and fear-based practice, as we know they do,[12] there is emotion work to manage our feelings and theirs.

Emotion work is the air we breathe as midwives. It's not just about internal conflict, it's what enables us to connect with parents and navigate our way sensitively through a labour, a change of circumstances or a situation of baby loss. The large amount of emotion work may be one of the reasons we chose this work in the first place. And yet high up on the mountains there is little oxygen left to tolerate the strain of the emotion work. Walking with a psychologist friend, she reflects on the similarities between her work and mine in terms of 'holding space' for intensity, vulnerability and deep transition. Her professional protocol and standard of excellence means she has one hour of clinical supervision for every eight hours of client work, in her case three times a week. She looks horrified at the thought of no defined or protected time for reflection and emotional support for midwives.

It's time to explore the mountains one by one.

# CHAPTER 4

# MEGA MOUNTAIN I: MORAL INJURY

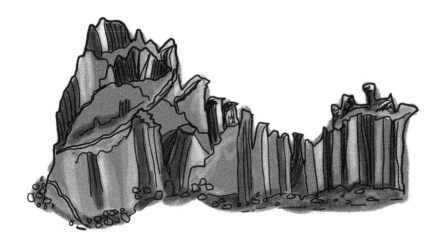

No one was really talking about moral injury before the 1990s, and it was first used to describe the internal experience of those exposed to war and hostile environments.[1] In a medical or maternity context we experience moral injury or moral distress when we are 'perpetrating, failing to prevent, or bearing witness to acts that transgress deeply held moral beliefs and expectations'.[2]

Doctors began to discuss it more publicly in the UK at the height of Covid-19 in terms of tortuous decisions over who was prioritised for care with a shortage of ventilators and staff.[3,4,5] Nurses expressed their horror and sadness (and the need to contain both) about people dying of Covid without the presence of their family. Moral injury shows up when we are unable to meet our foundational principle of 'first do no harm', or in midwifery terms, first be truly 'with woman' and her priorities, whatever they are.

It shows up particularly when external constraints lead us to prioritise tasks over human dignity – creating actions and feelings which are ethically insensitive or ambivalent. The inability to properly support the start of breastfeeding and build a woman's confidence because of the pressure to move her to a postnatal ward; denying entry to the partner of a woman in distress because current rules enforce separation; the vaginal examination which is 'due' at 3am even though the midwife suspects that this woman may be one of the approximately 10% of UK women with a childhood history of sexual abuse;[6] the vaginal examination 'due' at any time of day or night even though the evidence for their value as a tool of measuring labour progress is negligible.[7,8] A mechanistic provision of care would go ahead and do it anyway, which, even if carefully and sensitively done, creates sensations of disconnection from ourselves and from the families in our care, leading to deep dissatisfaction.

Chantelle came to midwifery as a mature student because she wanted to care for women and their families. Yet through her training, and days as a newly-qualified midwife, she had been quietly scaling down her vision of what it means to be a midwife, what's humanly possible. As a qualified midwife she increasingly experiences dissonance – that uneasy feeling of mental conflict that happens when her behaviours and beliefs do not line up. Cognitive and emotional dissonance creates stress and guilt, which makes her more vulnerable to burnout.[9] In response and as a smart coping strategy, she withdraws emotionally or switches off from women.[10] Families who experience her care feel the disconnectedness, and feel guilty and confused for 'being a bother',[11] at the same time as feeling disappointed or even angry that they can't get the care they need in their time of vulnerability.

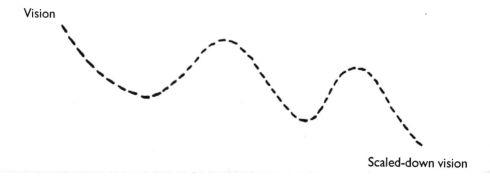

Vision

Scaled-down vision

## MIDWIVES ARE VULNERABLE TOO: DESPERATELY SEEKING 'SAFETY' FOR OURSELVES AS WELL AS FAMILIES

Have a look at this illustration of a midwife who is busy with the work of fulfilling institutional well-meaning policies or requirements, some of which have a thin or poorly justified evidence base. Look at the wedge her activity drives between herself and the family. Her chances of being able to give person-centred care are slim, and she knows it. There just isn't time when she has 'all this' to do. She justifies herself with the reasonable-sounding claim that she is busy preserving safety for the family. But she is just as much preserving her own safety in the moment: if all policies are followed and paperwork completed to the letter, then

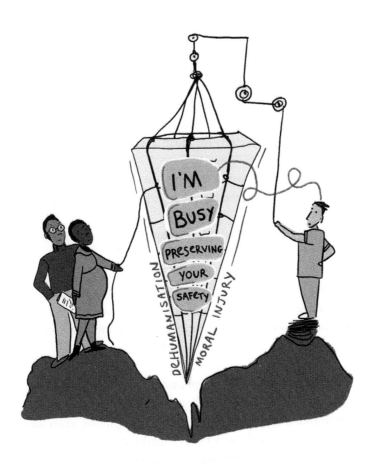

she is less likely, in the event of a bad outcome, to risk investigation and potential deregistration. She is finding herself having to put herself and the institution before the needs of the family, creating moral injury: a deep tension leading to dehumanised care and midwife burnout.[12]

We can all see the link here between ourselves and the families in maternity. When we as midwives learn or are pushed to give care that short-changes families – which takes the humanity out of our interactions – we and they are simultaneously dehumanised in the process.

> I am witnessing/involved in episodes of disrespectful care, birth trauma or coercion as part of my job.

> It hurts me because I can't completely protect these families. In 'leaving them' vulnerable I am overriding my most strongly held values. In that place, I too am vulnerable.

> I am a midwife. It is my role and my pride to be a 'guardian' of space, autonomy and dignity for these women and families.

> I want to be the midwife I signed up to be. I want to be 'with woman'. I should be protecting them and yet I am unable to do so.

> I know what is right, and what works for families (and colleagues) but I cannot do it.

> I feel some or all of these things: shame, guilt, powerlessness, frustration, overbearing sense of responsibility, lack of motivation, emotional distance from my work and the families, depression, spiritual crisis.

> I may behave in some of these ways: experiencing burnout symptoms such as distancing from the job or from my friends/family, drinking alcohol every day or to excess, hyper-exercising, becoming excessively busy or over-working as an 'avoidance' mechanism, self-harm.

Media reporting in 2020–21 around Covid and in 2021–22 around the staffing crisis in midwifery often used an image of a healthcare worker in scrubs crouched alone in a sterile corridor, head in hands. While the person is accurate (metaphorically crumpled even if we are not seeing it from the outside), the ultra-clean, unrealistically empty background smacks of confusion around healthcare: a wish for it all to be scrubbed clean, straightforward and therefore safe to enter. The reality is much messier – in heads and corridors alike. Another layer of mess – the plastic waste we generate – is also creating a form of moral injury, particularly among young cohorts of midwives horrified by the culture of extreme waste in maternity alone.

> 'It feels gross to be complicit in it; in a system which is so desperately behind in areas of sustainability and climate – and by extension social justice.' Katie, student midwife[13]

In 2021, the British Medical Association chose to survey doctors throughout the UK on the issues of moral distress and moral injury in the first pan-profession survey of its kind, prompted of course by the Covid pandemic, but not limited to it. As Deborah Morris says of moral injury in the 'Moral Matters' podcast, Covid just exposed what was already there.[14] Of the 1,900 respondents to the BMA survey, nearly half had not previously heard the terms 'moral distress' and 'moral injury', but were able via the survey to understand how much they reflect lived experience.[15] One participant said:

> 'I am so relieved to see these terms used rather than burnout or [physicians'] distress which imply only those with less resilience suffer from these "mental health" problems...'[16]

78.4% of nearly 2,000 UK doctors said that moral distress resonated with their experiences at work. 51.1% said the same about moral injury. 59.6% said they had been experiencing moral distress and injury well before the Covid-19 pandemic. Worryingly, although perhaps not surprisingly, given a background of systemic racism and the sustained micro-aggressions they see or face, doctors from

Black, Brown or Mixed Ethnicity backgrounds were more likely
to report that moral injury aligned with their experiences at work
compared with White doctors (64.6% versus 47.0% respectively).
Doctors with a disability or physical or mental health condition were
also slightly more likely to identify with a lived experience of the
term moral injury compared to those without a disability, although
the numbers in both groups were high (58.9% versus 48.4%).[17] Esther
Murray is embedded as a health psychologist at Barts' Health. She
has become a researcher and spokesperson around moral injury, and
has shown how the concept and reality also resonates strongly with
medical students who need opportunities to discuss what they have
witnessed and experienced.[18]

This overwhelming sense of recognition among health
professionals is probably not surprising. Our simplest moments of
enforcing or reinforcing so-called 'safety' can infringe not only on
our own values, but also on fundamental human rights – the right to
physical autonomy and integrity, for example, enshrined in Article
8 of the European Declaration of Human Rights, which is breached
every day by our failing to give sufficient, objective and unbiased
information to enable someone to make an informed choice,
including the right to decline any medical care at all.[19] Confronting
(and debatable) as that may sound, we are daily dealing with big
themes, whole lives and fully human rights. It is bound to take its toll.

## AN APOLOGY

*I apologise to you, bed 22.*
*I apologise because you're not a bed number, you are you.*
*You are a person with feelings, not just a medical condition.*
*You are a mum, growing a human, waiting to welcome your new*
*addition.*
*But you are an inpatient, something is not right,*
*And I'm trying, while you are here, to help you win this fight.*
*Be it blood pressure, sickness, or a baby who won't behave,*
*I see you there, waiting patiently, trying to be brave.*
*But you're scared; I can see that, you're out of your depth,*

*That's where we come in, to protect, to treat, so you can catch your*
*breath.*
*But we have other ladies, who also need our support,*
*In emergencies, in crises, not wanting their pregnancies cut short.*
*So in all this kerfuffle, you may slightly slip through the net,*
*But please know I'm thinking of you, wanting your needs to be met.*
*I know you're more than a bed number, more than part of the*
*wheel, a small cog,*
*But with all this going on, our brains can mist over with fog.*
*I'm just trying to prioritise, from one scared family to another,*
*And in reality, no one can juggle this many balls, no one has that*
*power.*
*I'm just one person; I am trying my best,*
*But it's not good enough, you shouldn't see our stress.*
*You should feel like an individual, not just a number,*
*Please know we don't think of you like that, It's just we are at risk*
*of sinking under.*
*We came into this job to advocate, protect and care,*
*And instead the system is making you feel invisible, like you're not*
*even there.*
*But when the day is over, and I go home at night,*
*I often call the ward, to make sure you are all right.*
*I hope the next midwife caring for you has a quieter shift,*
*So you can get the care you deserve, and ensure your needs aren't*
*missed.*
*So once again, I apologise to you, bed 22,*
*Please know that I know, you're not just a bed number, you are*
*you.*

Alicia Walker, midwife[20]

**What if** we could initiate an outpouring of honest feedback reflecting the interconnected role of the whole system and seeing the impact on *both* staff and families? How would this be?

A poster on the wall of the labour or postnatal room which asks 'How would you rate your midwife's kindness and communication?' And 'How has it made a difference to your ability to be kind to yourself or communicate well with your baby today?' With a quick-access online anonymous feedback space.

And one at the midwives' station saying 'How would you rate your team leader's kindness and communication?' And 'How has it made a difference to your ability to be kind and communicate well with women today?' With an online anonymous feedback space.

And one in the shambolic changing room saying 'How would you rate your department's kindness and communication?' And 'How has it made a difference to your ability to be kind and communicate well with women today?' With an online anonymous feedback space.

Real-time feedback is powerful and will set expectations for change.

## THE WOUND AND THE INFECTION: HOW MORAL INJURY LINKS TO THE OTHER MOUNTAINS

Moral injury is the wound, caused usually by the daily micro-transgressions where we step over the line of what we ourselves consider right, or are just part of the atmosphere that generates these decisions and actions. Burnout, or even post-traumatic stress, can be a manifestation, leading to a systemic infection which depletes all resources and often leads the sufferer to turn inward to survive.[21] And of course they overlap significantly. Support/treatment options are limited. The complexity of moral injury is partly due to sometimes overwhelming feelings of guilt and responsibility for having caused or not been able to prevent harm. Hannah Murray at the University of Oxford has been exploring using a cognitive therapy approach already validated for PTSD treatment for those exposed to moral injury.[22] Victoria Williamson, researcher at Oxford and King's Centre for Military Health Research, names the issue: 'Taken together, the international literature indicates that moral injury might be an important public health concern. Yet, no validated treatment for moral injury currently exists'.[23]

Back in the midwifery world, Patterson, Hollins Martin and Karatzias[24] focus on the need to acknowledge the harm caused by the system – the iatrogenic harm – on both sides of the relationship caused by poor care provider interaction (CPI). They call for positive CPI to be seen as more than a 'nice to have' – it is essential to the health and the safety of both families and midwives, and should be well supported and woven into the core framework of high standards in maternity.

I have pulled out a few of their recommendations as they are helpfully provocative. Notice how you feel about them, and see Part II to seize the opportunity to become part of the micro-shifts in this direction.

The researchers call for:

- An overhaul of midwifery tasks to remove unnecessary 'ticking of boxes'. *(I see you smile)*
- Meeting the physical and psychological needs of midwives and wider maternity care staff by prioritising time for support, restoration, and optimising the workplace environment.
- Developing, implementing, and evaluating an interpersonal skills toolkit for midwives.
- Urgently examining factors that prevent midwives having time with women, especially in the immediate postnatal period.
- Exploring midwives' wider needs, including from prior or work-related trauma, or mental health illness.
- Identifying and implementing organisational steps to meet midwives' wider needs.
- During obstetric interventions or emergencies prioritise midwives to *be with* women.[25]

As a newly qualified midwife, I remember feeling torn; pulled away from the birthing family in the midst of an assisted birth or emergency and pulled towards a task. Little explicit permission is given in skills and drills or PROMPT training (in a well-resourced environment) for a woman's midwife to be the one whose *sole* focus is kindness, touch and clear communication with a woman and family, which research shows minimises the risk of trauma symptoms, even in very challenging moments. This is also highly relevant to a transfer into the unfamiliar theatre environment, where the midwife's role is ostensibly to continue to be 'with woman', but definitely becomes 'with task'. A midwife friend of mine has counted: there are up to 25 significant tasks to be completed and documented in a short timeframe, very few of which involve any contact with the woman. 'Abandoning' and 'being abandoned' are twin strands expressed by midwives and women in research by Jenny Patterson and team in 2019.[26] Florence Wilcock, obstetrician and long-time advocate for a better maternity experience for families, mentions in 'The Midwives' Cauldron' podcast how this 'with task' position of the midwife in theatre betrays the birthing family at one of their most vulnerable moments.[27] What she doesn't mention is how it also betrays the midwife. See more in Chapter 16 about how to make this your one small project for shaking up the system.

## QUESTIONS FOR YOU: MORAL INJURY

- What do you recognise in yourself from this chapter?
- Think back to the last three episodes/shifts you found particularly challenging or draining. How was moral injury playing a part in your feelings or responses on that day or night?
- What, if anything, does this chapter inspire you to say or do?

# CHAPTER 5

# MEGA MOUNTAIN 2:
# COMPASSION FATIGUE

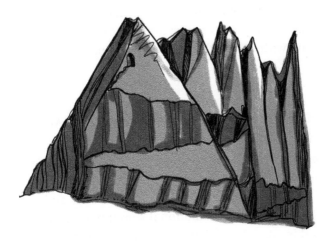

*'One day, you may realise how empty and lifeless your work has begun to feel. You're angry, depressed, or feeling numb. Maybe you dread your work, or you've turned into that bitter cynic you swore you would never become. Maybe you catch yourself dealing with fellow humans as though they were products on an assembly line. Maybe you can't find it in yourself to care anymore. Or maybe you're caught up in an unhealthy addictive behaviour.'*[1]

Sound familiar – even sometimes?

This is a description of what has commonly been called compassion fatigue. Agnes Otzelberger has lived in 'emergency' environments in the world of global development for more than a decade, and now studies the human response to working in professions that care and advocate for other humans/animals/the planet in the face of overwhelming challenges. She is using her experience to ask the vital question:

*'Is there a way to fully engage with suffering around us and in the world, and still feel the energy and joy we need to carry on with our work? Can we care AND stay sane, without looking away?'*[2]

The Schwartz Rounds[3] I facilitate, and which are facilitated in more than 500 healthcare sites around the world (one-hour reflective spaces designed to enable participants to engage with the emotional impact of caring), are there to support that same question. How on earth do we go on with this work, the joy and the pain, the dark and the light?

## WHAT MIGHT BE THE SIGNS OF COMPASSION FATIGUE IN MIDWIVES?

You will see below when we come to the 'naming dilemma' that there is considerable overlap between burnout, compassion fatigue and trauma exposure symptoms. Indeed, over and above the now familiar physical and emotional symptoms (headache, gastrointestinal issues, sleep disturbance, mood swings, irritability, depression, poor concentration and judgement), the most commonly cited symptom is emotional exhaustion and its effects on our personal lives.[4,5] The greater the emotional exhaustion, the more likely we are to use 'the silencing response',[6] which could play out at home or at work. At work, when emotionally exhausted, we might find the plaintive uncertainty or loud cries of a postnatal mother and baby, or the intensity of a woman in labour, difficult to be with. We might use pat answers to slip away quickly and minimise concerns, use humour to change the subject, feel angry towards them, fake our listening or give other kinds of 'half attention' autopilot responses.[7] I've certainly done this myself. And in my diminished state of empathy, I've added to my growing sense of disconnection from the meaning of my work by avoiding or retreating from certain people or situations, signalling with my eyes, body language, 1980s-style 'drugs round in progress' tabard or my too-sharp too-short words themselves that 'I have no time for you, I have no space for you.' Shocking and true.

You too?

At home I find myself intolerant to the strong feelings of my husband or children. There is no emotional room left in me for those feelings, all the emotional 'rooms' are full, signs flipped to 'occupied'. So I am likely to silence them too – by minimising, retreating or even turning away. I am unavailable. Naming this and staying connected through this takes careful negotiation and courageous conversations between couples or people sharing a household or a life. As midwives we don't talk about this enough.

What we certainly do is use hard-edged humour as a release valve. What's the only way to survive as a midwife? I love Agnes Otzelberger's description:

> 'When I wasn't feeling depressed about it all, I was feeling numb and in denial. I used to joke that the only way to survive working on climate change day-in day-out was to be a climate change denier. My options, it seemed, were to either "toughen up" or face emotional collapse. Occasionally, I collapsed. Most of the time, I toughened up. We don't get to cherry pick the emotions we shut out. The price we pay for being tough is high. Neurologically speaking, a selective numbing of our emotions is impossible. So with the pain, I shut out all the good stuff too, joy, elation, inspiration. Over time I became cynical, lost my spark, burned out.'[8]

## THE 'NAMING DILEMMA' – WHO CARES?

Compassion fatigue as a label has recently fallen out of favour. What was once termed compassion fatigue, as it might feel less pathologising for practitioners, but used interchangeably with secondary traumatic stress,[9] has been largely replaced by the term empathic strain or empathic distress fatigue. This change has its basis in new neuroscience.

What we tire of is not compassion, it seems, but 'affective empathy' or what Otzelberger calls 'our visceral, painful mirroring of others' suffering',[10] which can lead us to either emotional shutdown or emotional breakdown. This may be a surprise to some of us, as empathy is usually regarded as a backbone trait of midwives. But neuroscience seems to be revealing that empathy can be a trigger for either:

- empathic distress, an emotion which tangles us up with 'feeling with' the client and therefore is self-related and leads to stress, burnout and/or withdrawal
  or
- empathic concern/compassion, which is an other-related emotion, tending towards positive prosocial feelings and behaviour, and better health for the carer.

When neuroscientist Tania Singer used a brain scanner to explore empathy, she saw contrasting responses to images and sounds of human suffering. The control group showed elevated activity in the parts of the brain connected with pain and distress. By contrast, Matthieu Ricard's brain (French scientist and Tibetan Buddhist monk) lit up in an area linked with connection, affiliation and the love of a parent – he experienced profoundly positive emotions.[11]

So, much as we as midwives might be attached to the idea of being empathetic souls, and much as empathy is quoted by aspiring student midwives as a trait ideally suited for the long road ahead, the resonance it creates provides a stimulus. We then have to make a choice (by training our brains – see below) to choose empathic concern over empathic distress. Empathic distress is exhausting and unsustainable. As we slip into empathic identification with a woman in distress, we are likely to hear or feel some of the following: the sound of our own voice in our head strongly agreeing with her, a tightness across our chest, or a welling up in the eyes.[12] There is a sense of joining in or blending with her experience, which in my 10 years as a doula I often chose, and probably also glorified as the best for her, and a superpower of mine. The distinction I am making here is not about doulas and midwives, it's about the choice we all have to use activated empathy as a path to empathic concern – remaining connected with this person and absolutely desiring the best for them, without experiencing their emotions or trauma ourselves. Parents will identify with this need to differentiate between holding our own feelings of distress while practising the skill of differentiating ourselves from our child – while staying connected. Not always easy!

Alex Heath, Director of the TBR College of Perinatal Emotional Health, describes two helpful techniques she uses when she finds herself listening to a traumatic birth story and notices the signs of moving into empathic identification/distress:

> 'focus on your left foot, all four points or corners on the floor or in the sole of the shoe and keep repeating internally "left foot, left foot, left foot…" This allows the meaning-making, more emotional right-hand side of the brain to settle and helps to move you into the more logical left-hand brain – shifting into a more balanced state overall. On noticing that we are "joining in" consciously shifting ourselves emotionally away, not into disconnection, but into a place from which we can see ourselves as separate.' [13]

Alex then suggests repeatedly focusing every breath on breathing love and compassion towards this person,[14] an example of making use of the resonance of the empathy trigger to choose a compassionate response – compassionate to both parties – which then gives the energy to act.

As a student midwife I cared for a family in labour who were having their third baby girl. In a situation almost unimaginable in its horror and complexity, their second girl – a toddler – had died in a car accident during the pregnancy. As every twins and multiples midwife knows, it is a relatively common situation in midwifery to confront both the hope and joy of new life, and tragic loss, simultaneously. I acknowledged with the mother the death of her older child, and tried to hold the awareness of the gravity and beauty of the labour in the context of loss (while paddling away learning clinical skills along the way!). I advocated for them as a family when a shift in her labour threatened to expose her to more faces, more intervention. But as a student midwife I found this holding (and what I now recognise as my empathic distress response) overwhelming.

Alex Heath says:

*'I think "in the moment" it is natural for birth professionals to empathetically engage with birthing parents. It's such an intense process it would be hard not to join them at some points. I think it helps to realise that it is happening, which then enables us to move with or resist it, depending on what is best for us and the birthing parents. It also helps to acknowledge afterwards that the rinsed out, exhausted feeling is because of that empathetic joining – so that we can engage in activity to re-energise: resting, then re-engaging with a loved one, or some kind of caring for ourselves that facilitates a reset of the autonomic nervous system (massage, cuddles, talking, being in nature, etc).'* [15]

What a gift then, to me and to all of us, to be able to practise something really simple to help us to look suffering in the eye and stay present, and to make it less likely that we either collapse under the weight of it all or seek to run away from it.

It's called a *loving kindness meditation* or *befriending* and is made up of phrases to repeat to wish ourselves and other people well. It may sound a little weird at first, especially if you don't feel comfortable with the idea of meditating, but it can make a difference quickly. Neuroscientists Richard Davidson and Daniel Goleman, in their book *Altered Traits*,[16] took a deep research dive into how our wiring is affected by different meditation practices. They found that loving kindness meditation leads to incremental, lasting changes in our brains from the first few *hours* of practice and that the more we practise, the more stable compassion becomes as a trait.

You can find a link to the loving kindness meditation in the Resources Home section on p.231 under compassion fatigue/empathic strain.

Compassion here is a response which is fully emotionally connected, can be strengthened somewhat like a muscle, and unlike empathic distress or strain doesn't overwhelm us or deplete us. So if there is a way, neurologically speaking, to go on fully feeling, but in a healthier way, certain old midwifery/healthcare stories might need to be replaced with new ones. Let's try them out for size:

| Old story | New story |
|---|---|
| We just need to distance ourselves to look after ourselves | Emotional distance does not equal health self-care. It risks dialling down our other emotional responses – those of connection, joy, gratitude, creativity. |
| The problem is you are too empathetic/sensitive | Empathy/sensitivity itself is not the problem. We do need to be supported to learn to 'be with' our own empathy and with others' distress. Being properly in tune with our own and others' feelings is beneficial physically and psychologically. We can use our empathy response to trigger and grow our compassion response. |
| Self-care is the answer | Replace self-care with collective care so the burden of staying well is not on the individual. We can actively learn to expand our compassionate response when we find ourselves falling into trauma exposure responses, but we need to practice and reflect in our work communities to do it. Key message: this might require more than hot baths, time off and a sprinkling of yoga. Isn't this a relief? It's more like a Mount Everest expedition, requiring teamwork to overcome anticipated and real challenges and to prevent or delay the onset of altitude sickness (or in this case compassion fatigue or secondary traumatic stress) through open communication, mutual trust, interdependence, and strong team support.[17] |
| It's just the way it is; you have to learn to live with it | The human brain is not 'just the way it is' but an incredibly adaptive organ ripe for new connections |

## QUESTIONS FOR YOU: COMPASSION FATIGUE/EMPATHIC STRAIN

- Given your story, what are your particular vulnerabilities?
- How do you choose to protect yourself while doing this very challenging work?
- How have you come (at times or now) to realise that your work was having a significant impact on you and on your life?
- Where do the stories go? What do you do at the end of a work shift to put difficult stories from families or experiences with clients away before you go home?[18] (See Part II, p.199 for a transition from work to home exercise)
- What, if anything, does this chapter inspire you to say or do?

# CHAPTER 6

# MEGA MOUNTAIN 3: BURNOUT

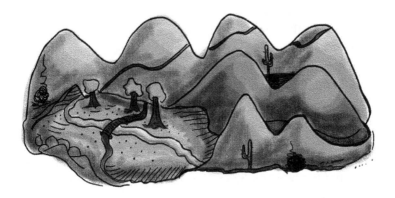

The phrase 'burnout', or 'burnt out', is often used in everyday language to describe exhaustion. In 2019 burnout was recognised by the World Health Organization in its International Classification of Diseases (IDC11) as a distinctly occupational phenomenon.[1] It is generally recognised to be gradually emerging, and a result of chronic workplace stress, but these definitions might also be helpful:

- *'A state of fatigue or frustration brought about by devotion to a cause, way of life, or relationship that failed to produce the expected rewards.'* Herbert Freudenberger, the psychologist who is attributed with coining the term 'burnout' in 1974.[2]
- *A state of physical, emotional, and mental exhaustion caused by long-term involvement in emotionally demanding situations.*[3]

Perhaps you recognise your own feelings or behaviours in these three key dimensions of burnout?

- *feelings of energy depletion or exhaustion;*
- *increased mental distance from your job, or feelings of negativity or cynicism related to your job;*
- *reduced professional efficacy and motivation.*[4]

At the end of my midwifery course, I found myself distancing from women in labour, choosing not to attend births – even the most potentially beautiful straightforward births – because of a feeling of not wanting to invest myself in the emotional energy required to be in that room. At the end of the degree and before I started work, for a period of about 6–8 weeks I didn't want to talk midwifery, read anything about midwifery or even talk to midwives other than my most trusted midwife friends, whose identity for me went way beyond midwife. And this from a woman who had been vociferously talking birth and advocating for families for nearly 15 years! It felt, in short, like the opposite of celebration and passion and anticipation. I was experiencing burnout. What compounded these feelings of not being myself was that the burnout itself was creating the confusion of prompting me to act against my own values, creating feelings of guilt and shame, and what I now recognise to be moral injury or distress. I value intimacy; I was seeking to avoid it. I value connection; it seemed like too much effort.

This distancing or disconnection as a symptom of burnout is obviously detrimental to both midwife and pregnant woman/birthing family. It is a connected relationship, after all, that both sides seek, and which can become a major source of satisfaction, safety and healing.[5] Given our distinctive role as midwives in promoting the emotional health of the mothers and fathers of the next generation, it is particularly terrifying to consider the impact, the missed opportunities, created by burnout in a maternity context.[6]

*'To be completely honest sometimes I just switch off a little bit and take a wee step back because I can't.'* Alice, midwife[7]

Billie Hunter's team investigating the extent of burnout and emotional distress among UK midwives in 2019, pre-pandemic, found that 83% of nearly 2,000 midwives reported moderate to high levels of personal burnout – impacting their personal lives – compared to 65%, 43% and 20% in the Australian, Swedish and Norwegian cohorts respectively. Two-thirds of the 2,000 had considered leaving midwifery within the last six months.[8] The 2021 NHS staff survey post-Covid shows the sharpest decline in job satisfaction among midwives compared to every other staff group, with particular concern around safe staffing – with only 6% of midwives saying that there are enough staff to run the service safely.[9] It shows dangerously low levels of morale among midwives in England, with 71% of midwives saying they find their work emotionally exhausting – nearly double the national average of 38%.[10] We don't often lift our eyes to see the wider picture beyond maternity, but the 2021 NHS staff survey reveals 63.1% of midwives regularly feeling burnt out because of their work, a score 12% higher than that of paramedics, and significantly higher than for nurses. A staggering 66.3% of midwife respondents said they have felt unwell as a result of work-related stress in the last 12 months, 20% more than the national average of 46.8% for NHS workers. This is a leap of 23% since the 2018 survey and a jump of 11.4% since 2020, in a period when the national average has only risen by 2.8%.[11]

A 2021 RCM survey of 1,581 midwives showed a staggering 57% intending to leave the NHS within the next year.[12]

It's easy to see how the effort and conflict of experiencing this:

*'I don't have time to connect to the women as individuals [...] I have increasing lack of compassion for women'*[13]

can turn into 'I just can't do it anymore'.

And because health professionals, including midwives, tend to be expert at emotion work and emotional labour – carrying on giving compassionate-looking care regardless of what is happening on the inside – these attempts to regulate their feelings on behalf of families and colleagues can increase the risk of burnout and can intensify emerging mental health problems.[14,15] 34% of UK midwives in a meta-analysis of studies were found to be experiencing at least moderate anxiety symptoms and 37% symptoms of depression, higher percentages than in the general population and higher than in midwives elsewhere in the world.[16] These numbers included and confirm the WHELM findings of UK midwives scoring in the moderate/severe/extreme range for stress (36.7%), anxiety (38%) and depression (33%).[17] This clearly has its consequences, on so many fronts. We see from Sally Pezaro's 2021 survey of 623 midwives that 28% were self-reporting persistent substance abuse as a direct response to work-related stress, anxiety, bullying and traumatic clinical incidents. 10% of the 623 said that they had come to work under the influence of alcohol and 6% under the influence of restricted drugs. 37% said that they were concerned about substance use in a colleague.[18] Persistent substance abuse has been identified in similar numbers in other populations of health professionals including nurses and doctors,[19,20] and has been linked, unsurprisingly, to occupational distress in paramedics.[21]

Midwife and writer Amity Reed's heart-wrenching account below details a common pattern of shame, isolation and fear of reaching out for help.[22]

*'I realised something was wrong when I began dreading going into work and found myself worrying about it endlessly on my days off, making it hard to relax and recuperate. Anxiety about whether I'd get to eat or rest during my shifts grew, as did the worry that I'd forget something or make a mistake because of how exhausted I was all the time. As a result, I began drinking alcohol more heavily in the evenings to try to help me switch off and sleep, which just made me feel worse the next day. I became more tearful and suffered horrible mood swings. Shame at my behaviour and what I perceived as my inability to cope led me to isolate myself from my family, friends and colleagues, until I found myself in a very dark, lonely place. The red flags started popping up everywhere, the biggest of which were crying upon waking up, feeling so sluggish that I could barely focus, heart palpitations, alcohol misuse, panic attacks and, finally, a suicide attempt.'*[23]

This is real, and it's going on all around us.

## A NOTE ON EXHAUSTION

Emotional exhaustion is a feature of burnout. Laura van Dernoot Lipsky, in her book *Trauma Stewardship*, describes this kind of exhaustion as a 'bone-tired, soul-tired, heart-tired kind of exhaustion – your mind is tired, your body is tired, and your spirit is tired.'[24] Many of us will relate to these descriptions of the impact of poor shift patterns:

> *'I don't remember the last time I had any energy and wasn't completely exhausted'*[25]
> *'so tired on my days off that I don't have the energy to do the things I want to do'*[26]

While it's difficult to separate physical and emotional exhaustion, it is true that in many medical environments, and perhaps particularly among doctors, exhaustion has become normalised and even championed as mildly heroic.

Exhaustion (there is no doubt about it) will bring distress. It takes us into the adrenal zone, where our adrenal glands are working overtime, attempting to maintain a state of alertness and vigilance, producing adrenaline for the perceived ever-ready fight, flight or freeze response focused on targeted immediate threats. We have been well trained for it – our bodies primed by an education system which encourages the adrenal response (and the activation of the sympathetic nervous system generally) with competition. But in this state, we lose our peripheral vision, our perspective, and therefore our ability to make good decisions. We tend to drive harder to compensate for the way we are feeling, compounding the problem. This persistent adrenal activity can manifest as symptoms of stress and

mental illness, including anxiety and depression. Dr Andrew Tresidder, on the 'You are not a Frog' podcast, points out that the lines between emotional exhaustion and anxiety/depression get very blurred. He emphasises the need to respect our mammalian physiology and deeply rest before any 'diagnosis' of mental health issues is made.[27]

A consultant obstetrician told me her story:

*'I had been working harder and harder, longer and longer hours to try and meet the requirements of the job. It simply never entered my head that what was being expected of me was unreasonable and unachievable. Instead I felt I was at fault for not juggling the many competing tasks successfully. I didn't realise there was a problem, I had no insight despite friends and family trying to tell me that I needed to stop. My body finally gave me the signal, it was only when I was in A&E in pain and I had stopped that I started to realise the difficulty I was in. I blamed myself for being unable to cope. I was feeling totally overwhelmed by work as if I was undertaking an assault course every day with no way out. My sleep was extremely disrupted, I couldn't get to sleep and when I finally did sleep I would wake up in the early hours and be totally unable to get back to sleep as I was wired. I spent many nights creeping out of bed and trying different techniques so that I wouldn't disturb my family. I spent a lot of time crying, I was exhausted. I was staying late at work and bringing work home, work dominated everything. I had written an email to my line manager saying my workload was unsustainable; this was initially ignored and then a month later acknowledged with a brief meeting in which I was told I did not know how to do my job. Eventually on sick leave, and in the aftermath of another punitive HR meeting to "manage" the situation, I considered throwing myself on the train tracks at the local station. I sat on a bench on the platform for ages.*

*I completely owe it to my occupational health department that I am still a doctor and was able to have a very gradual staged return. They were phenomenally understanding and helpful. I have learnt I need to set my own limits as to what I can and can't do and that it is okay to say I cannot do something. I still find this hard. I know that I am particularly susceptible to feeling over responsible for everything. I and my family are better at reading the warning signs, but I still struggle to call it early and protect myself sufficiently. I have learnt that teamwork is particularly important to me, belonging to a team and working with team members who can share responsibility and burden as well as supporting one another.'*

## WHO IS MOST AT RISK OF BURNOUT?

Burnout is common among all health professionals, including midwives. Some of the factors which predispose midwives to burnout are those that are blindingly obvious to us all – and they read like a horror show: 12–13 hour shifts in erratic patterns, pressured further by short staffing and extended by unpaid overtime, creating significant levels of physical and emotional exhaustion;[28] 87% of midwives reporting regularly having to delay going to the bathroom at work due to lack of time (I'm sure I'm not the only midwife grateful for a ready supply of oversized sanitary pads once a month); 75% of midwives reporting skipping meals, including more than 25% doing this almost every day; and over 50% of midwives reporting feeling dehydrated most or all of the time.[29]

The post shift(s) physiological hangover is real. Midwife Joanne Cull brings perspective from a former role outside of healthcare:

*'Before becoming a midwife, I spent a decade as a chartered accountant. Coming from that professional background, I was shocked by the way midwives were treated. I saw some managers making great efforts to arrange working patterns which suited the midwives in their team, and others who very much didn't. Similarly, I worked with fantastic coordinators that would make sure everyone got a break on almost every shift, and others where we rarely did. It's insanity to expect midwives to maintain focus and compassion for over 12 hours with no break. And we don't get paid for our breaks, so when we don't get them we're literally working an hour for free. Why was no one angry?'*[30]

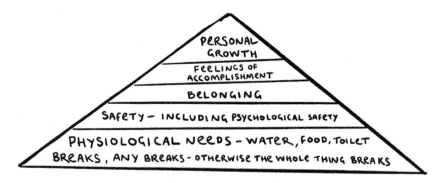

This model may be well worn, but it helps us to think again about the environments we are working in, what we need and what's missing. It presupposes that we require the fundamentals in the lower part of the pyramid to be in place – including having our physiological needs met – before we can progress to the headier heights of learning, growth and fulfilment. There has been much debate over the years about the intercultural applicability of this model. Some have argued that safety and belonging actually share the foundation of the pyramid with physiological needs, or that among a global majority, belonging/connectedness could also be seen to be the ultimate fulfilment of our purpose as humans.

What is clear, however, is that in many hospital environments even the most basic physiological needs of midwives are not being met. In fact, even the very existence of the long shift and the night shift is a physiological car crash. We simply can't overestimate the effect of nights on our physiology and emotional wellbeing, and we are only slowly discovering the true cost to health. Recent studies have confirmed the alarming impact of circadian misalignment. We now understand that almost all tissues in the human body exhibit cellular processes that align to a circadian rhythm and which synchronise to our 'master clock', stimulated primarily by light and dark. Misalignment by working and eating – especially eating a pile of white buttered toast – at unusual times leads to poor glucose and lipid tolerance, erratic insulin signalling, increased inflammatory markers and sluggish metabolism (night shift bloating is also real), all of which can contribute to the well-established risk of that 'midwifery spread' we all laugh about, type 2 diabetes, chronic sleep disruption and cardiovascular disease in shift workers.[31] It has been suggested that this is all made worse by the disturbance of our healthy gut microbiota caused by sleep loss and circadian misalignment.[32] And a recent meta-analysis stated that for every five years of night shift work, the risk of various common cancers increases by 3.2%: i.e. the effect is cumulative.[33]

And there's a hit for the predominantly female workforce in midwifery too: not only have female shift workers been shown to have a higher risk of developing metabolic syndrome and type 2 diabetes compared with male shift workers[34,35] (although a lower risk of hypertension),[36] menstrual irregularities, and difficulties with pregnancy/fertility, are also prevalent in the research, likely due to endocrine disturbance.[37] In a retrospective study of 128,852 women, night shift workers under 35 years old were more likely to require fertility treatment to conceive a first baby than their day shift counterparts, controlling for ethnicity, socio-economic status and smoking.[38]

Mental health is also heavily disrupted. Two recent meta-analyses have shown an increased risk of depression among night workers of between 33-42%.[39,40] It makes absolute 'sense' to all of us who have worked rotating, arrhythmic night shift patterns (that's *all* of us as midwives and student midwives), that disconnection from the daytime world of normality, light, friends and family, and the misalignment of all of our systems would increase the risk of depression and exacerbate the 'mountains' of midwifery we are also experiencing night by night – or night, by day, by night.

As Amity Reed says:

*'I started doing nights more because there was less bureaucracy and fewer managers and doctors to deal with, which was a big part of my frustration with the job. I felt like I could be more of a "proper" midwife on nights, but the toll it took on my sleep, family life and then eventually mental health was the price I paid for trying to carve out a bit more autonomy.'*[41]

We can see from the research data that night shifts and rotating shifts create higher burnout levels: midwives report higher scores for depersonalisation as well as low personal accomplishment.[42]

Depersonalisation creates an absence of psychological safety (to be discussed in Chapter 9), part of the second fundamental tier on the pyramid above, and an absence of belonging, the third tier. A sense of depersonalisation is probably not surprising given the common expectation that midwives rotate on a 24–7 rota, often part of a changing team, undermining a basic human need for connection and belonging.[43] This imposition of a rota organised around service needs rather than human ones can cause feelings of lack of personal control and autonomy over many aspects of our day-to-day work – a major contributor to stress and burnout.[44,45] NHS staff survey 2021 data[46] suggests that a significant proportion of midwives do not work in 'real teams', defined at a minimum as a small group sharing clear goals, and meeting regularly to review, reflect and improve.[47] Only 42.9% of midwives, for example, reported that they often meet to discuss their 'team' effectiveness.[48] For the estimated 50–60% of acute NHS staff working in 'pseudo teams', psychological safety is compromised by a lack of trust and inclusion, and is compromised further by pervasive pseudo-team-enhancing narratives of 'we're all one big team here'.[49]

There is good evidence to demonstrate that working in a supportive 'real team' with good leadership lowers levels of stress, errors, injuries, bullying and absenteeism for staff, and raises patient safety and satisfaction levels.[50] At its best, a team offers depth of relationships over time, co-responsibility for goals, and accountability to each other. The absence of a team can be a recipe for disconnection. Feedback and encouragement is harder to find in a rotational setting with fewer deep and trusting relationships. A sense of accomplishment might be achieved via getting through the tasks in hand, but it can feel like this midwife described herself:

> *'I am just a number, I do not feel valued as a midwife and it is all too much.'*[51]

Or perhaps even worse in the context of maternity care, as newly qualified midwife Ashleigh describes herself, 'just a body.'[52]

See 'Reimagining the handover' on p.114 to begin to address the issue of 'just a number'.

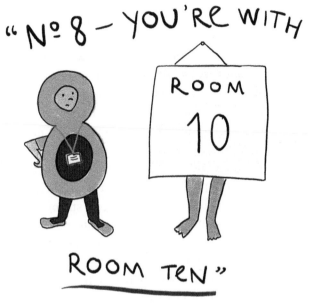

*Just a number meets just a number.*

## WHAT ELSE PUTS US AT RISK OF BURNOUT?

You may think this obvious, and we'll explore direct and secondary trauma in a later chapter, but exposure to traumatic events increases the chance of midwives experiencing burnout. 90% of the 137 Irish midwives responding to a 2020 study had been exposed to a traumatic event in the past year and 58% had been exposed monthly or more. The greater the distress, the greater the likelihood of burnout symptoms.[53] However, as Leah Hazard, midwife and author of *Hard Pushed*, points out:

> '"burnout" is not necessarily created by a sudden fiery blaze, but a series of burning fires over time.'[54]

Exposure to the kind of event which is not regarded by the system as major, adds incrementally to a midwife's sense of emotional exhaustion and moral distress – increasing the likelihood of burnout symptoms developing.

We explored the neuroscience around empathy a little in Chapter 5, but yes, shockingly, this trait that many midwives bring in spades, appears to also put us at risk of burnout.[55]

Finally, the WHELM study[56] identified the following groups as the most vulnerable to burnout and associated symptoms: midwives under 40 and midwives with less than 10 years' experience, particularly early career midwives in their first five years. Researchers have suggested that early career midwives' feelings of depersonalisation may be exacerbated by the need to focus on the task itself, the knowledge, the guideline, reducing the bandwidth to engage emotionally with the pregnant/birthing woman or person.[57] Early career midwives have also been identified as more likely to experience a strong emotional engagement with the family and an intensity of internal conflict as they seek to advocate for women in a system in which they are yet to establish themselves professionally.[58]

The susceptibility of early career midwives to burnout may also be because they are a group more likely to be working full-time, more likely to be subject to the lack of autonomy over hours in a rotational role,[59] more likely to be single, or less consistently supported, and less likely to have children. I can see you mothers of young children smiling wryly at the assertion that midwives with children are less likely to experience burnout. Perhaps it has something to do with the inevitable 'outside of work' life perspective of parents[60] and the pressing alternative focus that children create.

## WHAT CAN MAKE A DIFFERENCE?

It makes sense that the following will protect us as midwives from the slow hollowing of burnout:

*Personal and work autonomy, including independence over decision-making*
This is regarded as key and is found more in community than hospital settings.[61]

*Midwives' ability to actually be 'with woman' — linked to the autonomy above and to midwives' generally strong motivation to do the work*[62]
This is one of the reasons why (read my lips) well structured, fully

staffed, supported and funded continuity of carer models could still have the potential to reduce burnout.[63]

### Support from the employer for work-life-balance[64]

Self-rostering has been shown to help with a sense of autonomy and motivation.[65] This is an area which needs so much creativity and energy right now, as the cry of midwives to collectively create a better way is clear and pressing. It is easier to manage with a small to medium-sized team model, but remains possible with a rotational model. If you'd like this to be your micro-project for change, see Chapter 16.

### Connection

While exercise, of course, has a protective effect,[66] the NHS 5 Ways to Wellbeing number one below is actually *connection*. Exhaustion can be caused by loneliness and disconnection, and connecting with colleagues and team counterbalances this. Across an entire 13-hour day on a full postnatal ward with a new colleague, we managed to share half a sentence about our children/personal lives before being pulled into the next task. This is not how we are designed to work. This in itself is dehumanising. It is very clear from the research that strong team and colleague relationships are one of the main reasons midwives stay in the profession,[67] and that the camaraderie and humour and are a protective factor against the stress of the workload.[68]

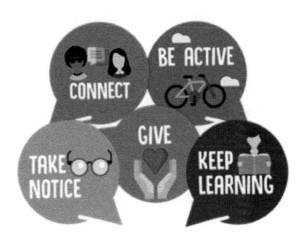

*Proactive behaviour* [69]

This is so easily underestimated. Joanne Cull gives an account of her proactive attempts to build in breaks and connection during long shifts:

*'I tried my very best to get a break on every shift. I always volunteered to take an early break, which meant I was more likely to get a break: lots of people would do the opposite and say they wanted a late break so the end of the shift went quicker, but if things got busy they didn't get a break at all. If I was working with a friend, I'd suggest we pair up to cover each other so we could both get something to eat and drink. When I was working on the wards, I'd suggest we all take a 20-minute break together and have a cup of tea, sometimes I'd bring biscuits. Lots of times it didn't happen, but when it did it was lovely.'*

Part II of this book is full of possibilities for experimenting with proactive behaviour on a micro and macro level.

Another aspect of proactive behaviour includes being given time to 'grow' the next generation of midwives. This is very significant and overlooked. It is reported as 'an affirming experience' by the midwives in Hunter and Warren's study on traits of resilient midwives.[70] This is not a side activity. As a nurturing profession, being given time to nurture our student and newly qualified midwives is an investment that reaps benefits for all. With an increase in the numbers of 18-year-olds entering midwifery courses as a consequence of the removal of the bursary in England in 2017, this is all the more necessary.

So, what is being designed or delivered in midwifery in terms of action on burnout? You would imagine that pre-emptive programmes of education and ongoing means of support to prevent and mitigate burnout would have been tried. Yet we know from the 2020 Society of Occupational Medicine report that very few primary intervention studies have been undertaken with nurses in the UK relating to burnout prevention and, to date, *no* initiatives have been implemented with groups of midwives.[71] Not one! There is work to be done! We do have the benefit of the POPPY programme[72] to mitigate against post-traumatic stress symptoms in midwives, which we will explore in

Chapter 8.

As you can see from the below graphic the strands of burnout, trauma and moral injury can't be disentangled.

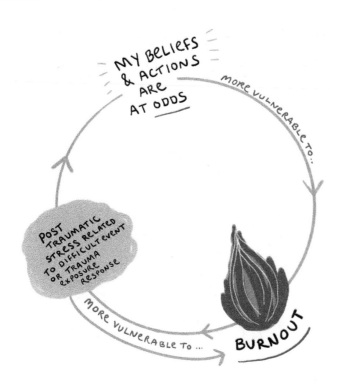

## QUESTIONS FOR YOU: BURNOUT

- Were you trained for this?
- How much were you made aware by your education or otherwise of concepts of burnout?
- What pattern of work would best protect you from burnout?

If you are currently experiencing burnout:
- Which of your values are currently being dishonoured/ disregarded? (see Part II, p.141 for an in depth exploration of your values)
- Who can you safely talk to or reach out to?
- What do you need now/next?

# CHAPTER 7

# MEGA MOUNTAIN 4: TRAUMA EXPOSURE

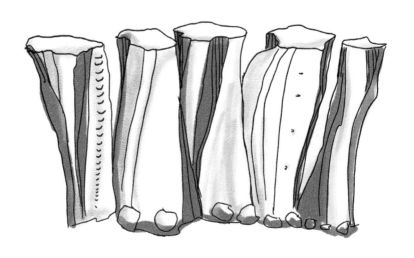

So let's talk about exposure to trauma – we can't ignore it any longer.

## TRAUMA EXPOSURE RESPONSE – POST-TRAUMATIC STRESS INJURY – SECONDARY TRAUMATIC STRESS

The focus of attention of maternity trauma research and advocacy has (you could argue rightly) been on the person giving birth experiencing loss or trauma. Researchers are now thankfully also turning the trauma spotlight on the midwives in the room, as human beings participating in and witnessing trauma. A small qualitative Australian study in 2013 was the first to explicitly do this,[1] with the first in-depth UK study of midwives' experiences as recently as 2015.[2]

## TRAUMA 101

We used to think of trauma as an event. And there *are* shock traumas that happen to us, like accidents, assaults and natural disasters. Mostly though, trauma is an experience not an event. It's about what we experience internally as a result of the ongoing story of our lives. This might be developmental or relational trauma if we have experienced chronic adversity, abuse or lack of safety while growing up; or our story might include other traumas like the experience of poverty, violence, discrimination, or – wait for it – chronic stress.

Stephen Porges's polyvagal theory takes us from a binary understanding of our nervous system between sympathetic (activated: fight/flight/freeze) and parasympathetic (rest and digest) to a more nuanced understanding of the fluid and flexible nature of a nervous system seeking homeostasis, moving up and down the 'ladder' backwards and forwards from a state of

- connection to others, effectively reading cues, muscles relaxed, to and from a state of
- activation of the sympathetic nervous system, organs and muscles responding to the need to fight or flee, to and from a state of
- shut down, a freeze state of immobilisation.[3]

While our autonomic nervous system (ANS) cleverly and involuntarily knows how to scan situations and people to determine if they are safe or dangerous and prompt us to react accordingly, background trauma can cause dysregulation of this system, so rather than functioning in a healthy way, the ANS keeps us stuck in survival. Our detection system becomes faulty, constantly signalling danger even when we are safe. In this state, we can't distinguish between our unsafe past and our now-safe present, and we replace our need for connection with our need for protection, some of which might play out in subtle immobilisation, emotional shutdown from the people we are with, or the environments and situations we are in. And because co-regulation with others who are safe, attuned and present is one of the best ways to help de-escalate our nervous system, high intensity, ever-changing environments like a labour ward are not always the most conducive to returning ourselves to a state of safety. Or in other words, environments like that can compound the trauma.

Are we seeing ourselves in this?

The third level, of immobilisation, the neurobiologically oldest and most primal state of the ANS, resonates strongly with survivors of trauma. In the scant research we have on midwives caring for women survivors of childhood sexual abuse, Lis Garratt draws a comparison between the dissociative (emotionally and mentally disconnected) state in the women, and a lesser but comparable dissociative state in the midwives, particularly in situations in which they felt powerless to act.[4] She says:

> *'Just as secondary dissociation provides survivors with a means of coping with the unthinkable, this [also] serves to minimise the emotional impact on the midwife and enables her to continue functioning. Instead of disappearing into a crack in the ceiling or a stain in the wallpaper, the midwife may focus on protocols, routines and rituals, thus disappearing into the system'.*[5]

I vividly remember my own feelings of confusion and even a sense of betrayal when, as a birth doula, I witnessed this emotional 'disappearance' or disengagement of midwives from the birthing family, most often when a birth was changing course, or as I now know, when a midwife under institutional pressure was choosing either consciously or unconsciously not to swim against the tide, but to dissociate from clients by focusing on the demands of the system.[6]

Emergency situations arguably provide another level of legitimacy for a midwife's disengagement. Lis Garratt quotes Sharon, a fairly newly qualified midwife, trying to explain what she found unexpectedly enjoyable about working in emergency situations on labour ward. She says:

> *'I don't know, maybe it's the rushing about. I don't know whether I take satisfaction in treating women with some degree of compassion and kindness and respect in dreadful situations, or whether the emergency side of it stops me having to emotionally engage with women...'*[7]

What a great question to be asking ourselves in relation to our own practice.

In fact, psychiatrist Bessel van der Kolk, in his work with veterans, and Lis Garratt in research with midwives, observed that a dissociative, numbed-out state can be so compelling as a survival mechanism that some soldiers, survivors, midwives and healthcare professionals only 'come alive' in the emergency moment, in the eye of the storm, in the midst of the drama.[8,9]

BBC war reporter Fergal Keane, who has made a recent documentary about his experience of PTSD,[10] conflict zone trauma surgeon David Nott[11] and Anna Kent, MSF midwife, recognise this pattern in themselves,[12] but it is also happening to colleagues in environments which appear far less extreme.

## WORK RELATED TRAUMA: BIG TRAUMA, LITTLE TRAUMA – IT'S ALL IN THE EYE OF THE BEHOLDER

*'Not all events that are perceived to be traumatic are objectively severe in their nature.'* [13]

We know this is true for pregnant and birthing women, people and families; it is true for midwives too.

There appears to be a wide spectrum of how midwives define work-related trauma for themselves. Descriptions of traumatic events include the expected and more visible events of death, injury, causing of harm,[14] mistake-making and exposure to acts of aggression from the family.[15]

However, a recent study of 170 Australian midwives[16] showed that they also included the following in their own midwifery experience of 'birth trauma':

- Witnessing disrespect towards women (including obstetric/midwifery violence or coercion in words or actions).
- Being disrespected as a midwife.
- Being part of poor care practice.
- Living with the ambiguity and knowledge that not everything goes according to plan.

- Conflict between models of care.
- Stress intensified by situational and workplace factors, one of which a UK study identified as limited or delayed access to resources or personnel.[17] This could be caused by staff shortages or by delays caused by poor communication or negative politics in the system. It also makes sense that the effect of the negative workplace factors is worsened when a midwife has a pre-existing relationship with the parents.[18] In her systematic review of women's and midwives' subjective experiences of care provider interaction, Jenny Patterson identified key research that showed that even in situations involving tragic outcomes, over and above the severity of the events, it was the interpersonal interactions that predicted PTSI in the women.[19] I wonder if the same might be true of trauma for midwives?

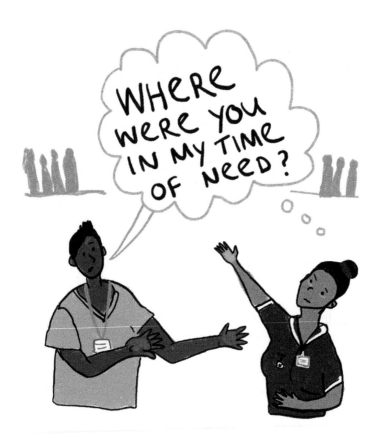

## MIDWIVES ARE VULNERABLE

All of these experiences increase midwives' vulnerability to trauma exposure response, post-traumatic stress injury and secondary traumatic stress.[20-23] A significant percentage (estimate 60%) of those entering caring professions have experienced some sort of primary trauma in the past.[24] Indeed, midwives will be represented (possibly over-represented?) in the 20% of the UK population with one adverse childhood experience (ACE), around 15% with two or three ACEs and around 10% with four or more adverse experiences as a child, involving violence, emotional or sexual abuse, neglect or substance misuse.[25] Midwives will also be among the 1 in 10 girls experiencing contact sexual abuse (by an adult) before the age of 16,[26] and the 7% of UK-based adult women experiencing domestic violence.[27] The strong trait of empathy among midwives, and the desire and expectation to be emotionally available to a woman, arguably also increases our vulnerability.

It all begs the question: why on earth aren't we working in a trauma-informed service – for us as well as for the families we care for?

In fact, researchers looking across the trauma spectrum are now strongly advocating for the midwifery profession to acknowledge traumatic stress as a professional risk.[28,29] This kind of evidence-based

---

**What if**, as we arrive at a university midwifery course or job interview, the disclaimer which currently says 'you will agree to work all and any hours God sends' also included the researched emotional and physical health risks of midwifery work and a warning that those who have the very skills and personalities that might make them most suitable for midwifery work are most vulnerable. What would it say?

And what if potential recruits to a maternity unit or team were to be encouraged to ask the following probing questions:
- how are you actively caring for your staff?
- what actions are you taking to recognise, talk about and help with staff trauma exposure?

---

information on entering the midwifery profession would also enable potential recruits and students to choose practice environments or employment wisely, and explore our personalities in relation to the risk to us. That is, after all, the kind of informed decision-making we claim to espouse.

Hopefully the widely viewed scenes of post-traumatic stress injury played out in the BBC adaptation of Adam Kay's *This is Going to Hurt*[30] will stimulate some honest conversations about what is urgently needed for maternity staff.

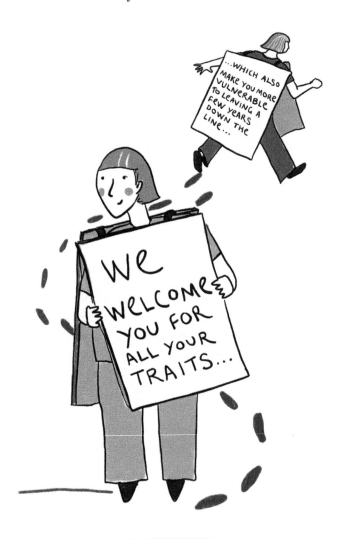

## TRAUMA EXPOSURE RESPONSE: IT HAPPENS OVER TIME, IT'S TO BE EXPECTED – BUT IF WE ARE AWARE WE CAN ACT TO MITIGATE THE EFFECTS

While 'post-traumatic stress' may conjure up graphic images of the battlefield (midwives will laugh with black humour about the similarities), what we as midwives are likely to be experiencing more *consistently* is ongoing trauma exposure, including being involved in difficult events or the difficult lives of families we care for, hearing about traumatic events or situations, or witnessing or supporting colleagues who are experiencing suffering. From this, a so-called 'trauma exposure response' may emerge. This shows itself in more subtle ways in our bodies and minds than post-traumatic stress injury.

Laura van Dernoot Lipsky works with people whose jobs are in some way trauma-exposed – from working in healthcare, to social work, to trying to minimise environmental destruction. She identifies 16 consequences or 'symptoms' of trauma exposure.

It may be that you personally identify with one or more of these signs of trauma exposure response – or you have seen them playing out in others around you in the midwifery world. The changes in you, if any, will be a clever adaptation to help you manage or survive your environment. Those changes could show anywhere on a continuum from slight to dramatic or life-changing.

As van Dernoot Lipsky says in *Trauma Stewardship:*[31]

*'For many of us, the elaborate architecture we build around our hearts begins to resemble a fortress. We build up our defences, but the trauma keeps on coming. We add a moat, we throw in some crocodiles, we forge more weapons, we build higher and higher walls. Sooner or later, we find ourselves locked in by the very defences we have constructed for our own protection. We will find the key to our liberation only when we accept that what we once did to survive is now destroying us. And thus we begin the work of dismantling our fortress, releasing the crocodiles back to their habitat, and melting down the weapons to recycle into plowshares. Rather than fend off life, we slowly train ourselves to open our hearts to everything that comes to the door.'*

I've included all of the below descriptions partly just to highlight how a gradually accumulating trauma exposure response can take such a lot of joy, curiosity and creativity out of our lives. And how – because it happens gradually – it can be so difficult to spot or to disentangle from the impact of current events in our everyday lives. Indeed, it may not have even occurred to us that some of the pain/events/stories we experience at work can actually change our own psychological and physiological responses, altering our worldview.

It's also important to say how hard it can be to look honestly at how our stance on the world is being affected by our work culture and what we're exposed to. See how *you* feel as you read through these signs and their attached questions. Go ahead and circle or place a question mark next to the ones you see in your life right now. Then challenge yourself to do it again, read it slowly, and notice where there are signals in your body that some of this might be happening for you. And remember that *not* identifying with any of these as trauma exposure responses may not necessarily mean they are not there, just normalised! Isn't this fun?

## Minimizing

- Does it take a more intense level of suffering to get your attention?
- Do you consider less extreme experiences of trauma for you or others 'less' real and therefore less deserving of your time and support?
- Do you downplay anything (often with humour) that does not fall into the 'most extreme' category of event?

## Chronic exhaustion/physical ailments

- Do you believe that you have very little choice about the work that you do?
- Does your workplace culture imply that fatigue is an accepted aspect of the seasoned worker's demeanour?
- Do you have a bone-tired, soul-tired, heart-tired kind of exhaustion – your mind is tired, your body is tired, and your spirit is tired?

## Addictions

- Do you use alcohol, drugs, cigarettes, or other distractions like phone scrolling, to check out?

- Are you addicted to the rush of adrenaline?
- Do you have a desire to stay wired so you don't have to slow down and really feel what is going on within and around you?
- Are you working most of the time, perhaps responding to urgent requests from an over-stretched workplace?

## Hypervigilance

- Do you often feel like you are always 'on', even in times where nothing can be, or should be done?
- Are you so focused on your job that sometimes being really present for anything else in your life can seem hard?

## Sense of persecution

- Do you have feelings of profound lack of efficacy in your work and/ or life?
- Have you become convinced that others are responsible for your wellbeing, and that we lack the ability to transform our circumstances? ('If only they…, then…')

## Sense you can never do enough

- Is there a feeling of urgency in the workplace?
- Do you ask yourself: Am I good enough? Tough enough? Clever enough? Do you believe you are not doing enough and you should be doing more?

## Feeling helpless/hopeless

- Do you frequently ask yourself if you are making an impact?
- Do you ask yourself what's the point?
- Is it difficult to see that any progress is being made for a positive change?
- Do you feel overwhelmed, as if nothing can remedy the situation?
- Are your successes hard to keep in focus, either in the day-to-day or in the big picture of your life?

## Difficulty embracing complexity

- Do you participate in cliques, gossip, and have rigid expectations of other workers or women/families?

- Do you crave clear signs of right and wrong; good and bad – while feeling the urgent need to choose sides?
- Are you more likely to say 'no', and be more opinionated?
- Do you look to take a side in a debate no matter what the debate is about?

## Grandiosity

- Do you feel that your work is so incredibly important?
- Do you ask yourself who else would/could do this job if you weren't here?
- Is work becoming the centre of your identity?

## Inability to listen/avoidance

- Is the highlight of your workday when you don't have to do your job?
- Has avoidance begun to show up in your personal life?
- Do you avoid answering phone calls?

## Guilt

- Do you ever feel guilty about finding things in life pleasurable when clients/colleagues you work with are suffering?
- Does guilt distract you from being present in your life?

## Dissociated moments

- Have you lost track of moments in your work because something someone said has unhinged you?
- Do you have difficulty staying present?
- Do you ever forget the last five sentences you have spoken, or find yourself not hearing the last part of what someone has shared?

## Anger and cynicism

- Do you know how your anger looks to others/your support system/ your partner?
- Is your humour in the workplace responsible or cynical? (A cynical sense of humour can be an effort to cope with anger.)

## Inability to empathise/numbing

- After becoming overwhelmed do you have difficulty experiencing any type of emotion? Regulating emotion?

- Do you find yourself crying disproportionately at a TV advert or raging at the dog/colleague/family member?
- Do you have numbed out intense feelings because you are scared and feel out of control?

## Fear

- Does bearing witness to the suffering of others bring to light the dangers of the world?
- Do you have a fear of intense feelings or personal vulnerability?

## Diminished creativity

- Do you get bored with what you're doing in your work?
- Do you feel stagnant in your ability to be innovative?
- Are you experiencing a decrease of joy in your life?
- Do you actually crave more structure and less creativity?

(Adapted from: Jennifer Froh, Juneau County Health Department. Original content from: *Trauma Stewardship: An Everyday Guide to Caring for Self While Caring for Others*. Laura van Dernoot Lipsky with Connie Burk; Berrett-Koehler Publishers, 2009)

## THE IMPACT OF A FEAR-BASED CULTURE

A trauma exposure response is of course heightened by working in (and absorbing the values of) a fear-based culture. We have already touched on the fear of litigation and deregistration prevalent in midwifery storytelling. Those *big* fears are part of a food chain of fears. We might ask the question: how does focusing on what could go wrong actually prime us for experiencing trauma?[32]

> 'I am constantly on alert and check the procedures just in case. I have become a code-red thinker. Being a midwife is dealing with critical incidents waiting to happen.' Midwife, 2020[33]

Minooee et al, in 2021, chose to explore in depth with 25 Australian midwives the question of whether this kind of fear-based thinking – so called 'catastrophic thinking' – is in fact the legacy of experiencing traumatic births. They specifically explored the impact of episodes of shoulder dystocia on midwives' feelings and clinical practice around physiological births.

They describe a shift, a disturbance[34] in these midwives, even after just one episode of shoulder dystocia, from a focus towards straightforward birth to one of hypervigilance. Interestingly it was the midwives' strength of relationships – both with women and colleagues in a continuity of carer model – that appears to have lessened the impact of the trauma, reduced the chance of PTSI symptoms, and enabled the midwives to maintain an equilibrium in the way they practise.

It makes sense that a distinct team, with time together at some point after an event, would be able to focus in informal, helpful ways not just on the event, but also on the feelings and emotional repercussions for the midwife. It also makes sense that a natural connection with the family involved would mean that the midwife could reconnect with the family, and have sense-making conversations which might help mitigate the trauma on both sides.[35] The majority of midwives, still working fragmented shift patterns with different colleagues every day and unknown families to care for, are therefore at even greater risk of an ever-deepening fear-based model of thinking, and the trauma exposure response that may follow.

Remember that a changed worldview, or the 'symptoms' of a trauma exposure response listed above, can respond to healing – see Part II to experiment with exercises to reshape your view of yourself in the world and develop strategies in your mind and body to soothe and soften.

## WHAT ABOUT SECONDARY TRAUMATIC STRESS (STS) OR VICARIOUS TRAUMA (VT)?

While secondary traumatic stress is sometimes used in the literature to describe the second victim directly experiencing or witnessing the trauma of another,[36] STS is more commonly used as a way of describing the response of those experiencing a traumatic event 'second hand' or indirectly, especially when 'helping or wanting to help'.[37] The words vicarious trauma are also sometimes used to describe the accumulation of this kind of indirect trauma:

*'the transformation* [or you could say contamination] *of our view of the world due to the cumulative exposure to traumatic images and stories'.*[38] (Words in square brackets mine.)

This could occur via a multitude of midwifery situations, including:

- Reading case reports of women experiencing domestic violence.
- Caring for vulnerable families who have experienced a history of trauma and hearing details of their stories.
- Being involved in FGM support and listening to stories of family betrayal and helplessness in the woman or girl.
- Having colleagues recount to you the graphic details of a traumatic birth (whether in a so-called 'debrief' or just because you happen to be there).

Mollart, Newing and Foureur[39] looked at the impact on midwives of conducting structured antenatal psychosocial assessments with women – using screening and assessment tools for domestic violence, childhood trauma, drug and alcohol use, depression, and vulnerability factors. They describe a cumulative emotional effect, with few support systems for midwives, and some midwives using unhealthy ways of coping with overwhelming feelings of frustration and vicarious traumatisation.

Canada-based Françoise Mathieu, a pioneer in 'helping the helper', describes these experiences and stories as the ones that seem to 'hitch a ride with us' after hearing, seeing, or reading about them.[40] Midwifery, as I said in the introduction, is a profession of storytellers. It is one of the ways in which female knowledge has always been passed on; 'herstory' told through generations and via community 'handy women' prior to the so-called professionalisation of midwifery in the early 1900s.[41] It is also one of the ways in which we as midwives 'process' the uncomfortable edges of our work, and the absurdities of the environments we work in. And it can get messy and be harmful.

## STORY SLIMING

How many times have you heard midwife colleagues recounting 'war stories': times when a woman was 'hosing' blood? What kind of image does that leave in your mind? Actually, often you will hear the phrase in this context: 'luckily she *wasn't* hosing', leaving the same imprint, even though it is phrased in the negative and an expression of relief, and also betraying how strong the (understandable) fear of excessive rapid blood loss has become; how much of a totem it has become of perhaps the ultimate fear of maternal death in our care. This kind of storytelling easily creates hyperarousal in the listener around the time after birth and birth of the placenta, already an acutely sensitive time for the birth family and a highly attentive time for a midwife.

Mathieu asks these very helpful questions to challenge us to reflect on our storytelling:

- How much we might have got used to debriefing informally 'all over' our colleagues? What is the context in those moments?
- Do they (or you, if the situation was reversed) have a choice to receive it or not?
- Can we even properly debrief if we *don't* share all the graphic details of a trauma story?

She shares the helpful strategy of 'low-impact debriefing': giving fair warning, asking for consent, and managing the disclosure in terms of content and pace.[42] Using this approach gives us greater choice: we can balance our natural curiosity about people and their stories of life and birth with what we now know could be healthy or unhealthy boundaries for ourselves or others. We can experiment with avoiding adding to the cycle of secondary traumatic stress of vicarious traumatisation, while at the same time more closely identifying what we need when we have heard or seen hard things. See more detail and encouragement to practice low-impact debriefing in Part II, p. 205.

## WHAT DOES SECONDARY TRAUMATIC STRESS/ VICARIOUS TRAUMA LOOK LIKE?

When associated with a particular event or story, it is possible for symptoms of STS to develop rapidly and mirror symptoms of post-traumatic stress, including midwives experiencing intrusive images, intense fear or feelings of helplessness and sleep difficulties.[43] When experiencing STS a midwife's instinctive response might be to avoid triggers linked to the story and to withdraw from the emotional intensity of relationships with families – the kind of 'empathic identification'[44] which in turn saves to protect a childbearing family from trauma. This potentially creates a vicious cycle of the midwife feeling dissonant or 'out of sorts' with herself, giving 'emotionally distant care',[45] thereby increasing both woman and midwife's risk of ongoing trauma exposure. However both STS and VT come under the wider umbrella of cumulative trauma exposure response (See pp. 80-83 for common signs of a trauma exposure response).

*'I used to enjoy being in the flat on my own with my two [young] boys at school. I used to love the silence. Now I have to have Netflix on in the background even though I hate Netflix... I can't be with the stories in my head.'* Midwife, one-year post-qualification[46]

*'I've started drinking every night. Just a glass or two. Just something to quieten the feelings, the noises...'* Newly qualified midwife[47]

## QUESTIONS FOR YOU: TRAUMA EXPOSURE

- What do you recognise of yourself in the words of this chapter?
- How are you beginning to see how trauma exposure is shaping you?
- What action will you take or conversation will you choose as a result of your growing awareness?

# CHAPTER 8

# MEGA MOUNTAIN 5: POST-TRAUMATIC STRESS INJURY AND THE BRAIN

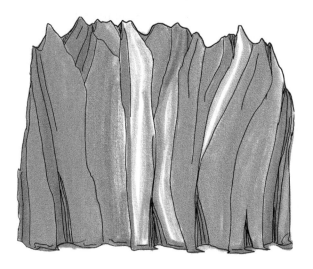

Post-traumatic stress injury is an occupational hazard.[1-3] Language is powerful: notice your own response to my choice of the word 'injury' here rather than 'disorder'. How does the responsibility shift between the use of those two words? The researchers who proposed this shift in language suggest we consider referring to post-traumatic stress as an injury (PTSI) rather than a disorder (PTSD), shifting the focus from the individual (the problem that I am experiencing) to the system (what is being done to me/what I am being exposed to).[4]

It is easier to research and measure the bearing of traumatic events on a clinical or subclinical diagnosis of post-traumatic stress

(American Psychiatric Association DSM-V), rather than gradual trauma exposure, so much of the research on midwives and health professionals has focused on PTSI (usually called PTSD).

In a 2015 survey of UK midwives with 421 responses, 33% of midwives reported symptoms of PTSI after being exposed to traumatic perinatal events involving a perceived risk to the mother or baby which elicited feelings of fear, helplessness or horror in the midwife. 5% of midwives had scores in line with a clinical diagnosis of post-traumatic stress.[5] The authors regard these percentages as conservative estimates of the number of midwives affected. Other studies bear out the high numbers of midwives experiencing symptoms indicative of post-traumatic stress or secondary traumatic stress injury,[6,7] including a 2022 systematic review including 8,630 maternity health professionals. This concludes that between 45% and 97% of maternity staff have been exposed to traumatic birth events, with the prevalence of STS ranging from 12.6%-38.7% and the proportion of participants meeting diagnostic criteria for PTSI ranging from 3.1% to a shocking 46%.[8]

Joanne Cull, midwife and researcher, shared her story:

'When I started my midwifery training, I was stunned by how cold some of the midwives and doctors were. Although I was pleasant on the surface, I judged them for what I perceived as lack of empathy towards the women in our care. Near the end of my preceptorship, I cared for a woman whose baby died in early labour. This was a terrible, terrible experience and in the aftermath I was a nervous wreck at work. If I couldn't pick up the fetal heart rate straight away, I would be convinced something awful had happened. More than once, I would keep my composure in front of the parents, then burst into tears as soon as I left the room.

I was touched by the sincere support I received from some of the same midwives and doctors that I'd judged so harshly. When they shared their own experiences with me, I was deeply troubled by what they'd gone through, often with very little support. Penelope Campling has written beautifully about the huge challenges which face NHS staff as they muster "the necessary

*balance of kindness and professional detachment."[9] Campling*
*suggests that lack of space and support to process feelings of*
*emotional trauma leads to defensive coping styles and reduced*
*capacity for empathy.*

*Midwifery is heavy emotional labour, and this is compounded*
*in the UK by a decade of neoliberal healthcare reforms which*
*prioritise cost-cutting. We're just beginning to understand how the*
*pressure midwives are under affects them.'*

Others in maternity are of course not immune. In a 2020 survey of
1,095 obstetricians via the RCOG, followed by 43 in-depth interviews,
two-thirds reported exposure to traumatic events, with 18% reporting
clinically significant symptoms of PTSI, and 32% experiencing subclinical symptom levels, with serious work and home-related impact.
91% wanted a system of care to mitigate the impact of events like
this, which would hopefully reduce the heartbreaking 30% of trainee
obstetricians leaving during their seven-year training. Black, Brown
and Mixed Ethnicity staff were found to be at increased risk of PTSI.[10]
See more on the reasons for this below.

## WHAT IS THE IMPACT OF POST-TRAUMATIC STRESS ON MIDWIVES?

We know from in-depth interviews with midwives after traumatic
events that midwives experience emotional exhaustion including
sadness, flashbacks, guilt, fear and intense empathy for the family
involved. Defensive practice becomes common – midwives protect
themselves from the accusation of even the smallest amount of
'risk-taking'[11] having focused so closely on the woman's feelings
and laboured intensively over the question 'What could I have done
differently?'[12] even if the answer is nothing. Indeed, being told
'there is nothing you could have done differently' doesn't actually
make the difference you might expect. Strong feelings of blame,
shame and vulnerability make asking for genuine help even more
difficult, especially in work cultures where traumatic events are
normalised, as it would mean admitting to these confusing feelings.[13,14]
Unsurprisingly, symptoms of post-traumatic stress in midwives are

associated with more negative perspectives on the world and feelings of burnout.[15] In her work on the relationship between midwives and women who have experienced childhood sexual abuse, Lis Garratt comments on the relative ease with which she observed midwives moving into a state of dissociation when witnessing a traumatic event and feeling powerless to act: 'displaying an amazing degree of detachment, apparently rendering them oblivious to the distress of others'.[16] As she points out, dissociation has strong links with post-traumatic stress disorder (PTSD) and can occur in any situation in which the person feels helpless when extreme emotions such as fear, terror or horror are evoked.[17]

## THE SECOND VICTIM IS YOU (OR ME)

Look how stark (and familiar) a common trajectory is for the 'second victim' of an incident – much of which can compound rather than alleviate the trauma, with re-triggering events and absence of help when it is most needed.

### Trajectory of recovery for a second victim

*The event is recognized*
*Sense of confusion, panic, concentration difficulties*
*Activities all about managing the woman/family*
*Midwife involved begins to comprehend magnitude of event*
*Midwife experiences flashbacks*
*Midwife experiences self-doubt*
*Loss of confidence in professional skills and identity*
*Mulling*
*Search for acceptance*
*Need to regain trust from colleagues*
*Worry others may not understand*
*Multiple episodes of recounting the event during organisational investigation process*
*In-depth case review*
*Triggering*
*Sense of apprehension over future employment*

*Concern over loss of PIN/registration*
*Midwife seeks emotional support, but where to find it may be*
*unclear*
*Emotional support may be unavailable*
*Trust issues: who is safe to talk with?*
*Silent suffering*
*Healing may begin*
*Possible outcomes: dropping out, surviving with lingering scars,*
*thriving...*

Adapted from McDaniel and Morris, 2020[18]

Dr Ruth-Anna, quoted in *Nurturing Maternity Staff* by Jan Smith,[19] admits that in her first decade of work as an obstetrician, she had never heard the term 'second victim', until a significant event took place on a bank holiday night shift when she was unwell, exhausted and early pregnant herself. This, and the subsequent process, following a similar pattern to the one above, put her at risk, just like many midwives, of telling herself that she was 'not cut out for this'. The truth was so different: she was suffering from a traumatic incident as the second victim, another person afflicted by intensely visceral flashbacks and feelings of fear and helplessness as a result of an event she herself experienced as traumatic.

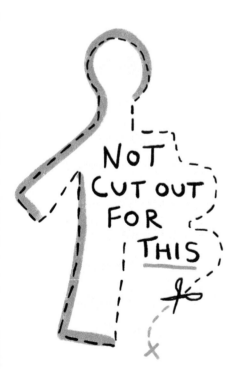

NOT CUT OUT FOR THIS

## TRAUMA AND THE BRAIN

PTSI is not inevitable. But experiencing or witnessing trauma does require rapid access to trauma-informed and focused psychological intervention in order to protect the person from potential longer-term effects.

Peter Levine has spent a lifetime developing body-based approaches to traumatic events. It is clear from his work that being able to come back into our bodies immediately after a traumatic event is a game-changer: we have to create a feeling of enough space and safety for people to experience the physiological shock itself (including helpful shaking, trembling, changing blood pressure, etc) before we can deal with any emotions – let alone try to access verbal processing of what happened or what it all means.[20] Going back to Stephen Porges's polyvagal theory this makes sense: whether the person is locked in the fight/flight or freeze response they are functioning primarily in the brainstem, and the language of the brainstem is the language of sensations. So if you are trying to help the person in that moment to mitigate the impact of the trauma (and also later in therapy), you have to talk to that level of the nervous system. Peter Levine has called it bottom-up rather than top-down processing.[21]

In the immediate aftermath of an event we go into a childlike state of feeling completely unprotected. We need direct contact with someone who is trauma-informed enough to know that they can't 'make it better', distract us, talk about 'it', rationalise or succumb to any other tempting human instincts. Instead they can either just be there with us or use something called verbal first aid. Judith Acosta and her colleague Judith Prager, in their book *The Worst is Over*, have shown the powerful effect of verbal first aid on the autonomic nervous system because, in the midst of a traumatic experience, we are in a suggestible state.[22] Scripts and pacing skills (of benefit to birthing families *and* maternity staff in and after the moment) could be learned by colleagues in mandatory training, backed up of course by a trauma-informed system with structures that support the second victim. Scripts might read something like 'The worst is over... I am here with you now... I'm not going anywhere and there is nothing else to do now... Except be fully in your body, feeling and allowing all that's there...'

Levine describes himself on the pavement after a car accident when, because of a kind paediatrician passer-by who sat down next to him and held his hand, he was gradually able to actually experience the sensations of what had just happened in his body as micro movements, which created an unexpected strength in his body. Minutes later, in the ambulance, as he let himself re-experience those movements and let his body shake and tremble (an important and helpful resetting of the autonomic nervous system) and feel the different emotions including visceral rage at the woman who had hit him, he was able to ground the sensations in his body and his blood pressure completely normalised.[23] This grounding in the body is in stark contrast to the common experience of a traumatised person frozen in immobilisation/fight or flight, frozen in a bodily reaction to the event, often literally contracting muscles to respond to danger, which can create chronic illness or pain, with or without PTSI. The basic principle is that if we're able to reset our physiological system, able to reset our nervous system, then we can avoid or mitigate the symptoms of trauma.

This calls for a new, shiny, soon-to-be-blood-spattered laminated poster in the manner of a sharps injury poster in the sluice. Everyone vaguely knows what to do when they get a sharps injury... encourage the wound to gently bleed, under running water if possible. Wash hands with soap and water and do not scrub the wound, do not suck the wound, get help with prophylaxis. Above all *don't not act*.

Actually, in the moment we often can't remember exactly what to do, as we generally feel pretty embarrassed and stupid, but the poster – and the compassionate education around it – helps remind us. Find a visual version of the poster below, customised for your maternity unit, at www.flourishformidwives.com/trauma-poster.

---

**What if** we were to offer the same automatic, expected and compassionate response for trauma exposure?

## JUST BEEN EXPOSED TO TRAUMA?

**Normal feelings now**
First know that you are going to feel overwhelmed, guilty, angry (if you've seen poor practice or felt under-supported), scared of the implications or intensely sad for the family involved. You might also feel completely numb. Whatever you are feeling, let it be there. And as much as possible try to feel all that you are feeling in your body. A cup of tea with sugar is helpful, but not the solution. And words of reassurance are not going to work right now. Ask for someone to be with you with whom you feel safe and can just be, with no expectations.

---

**Your wise brain and its strategy**

For the next month or so, your brain will be seeking to sort through what happened and will bug you with images you don't want to see and memories you would rather never recall. It will even stir them into your dreams at night. Triggers for intrusive thoughts might be simple, sensory and unavoidable – smells, textures, sights and sounds. They will come without warning and knock you sideways. This is horrible, and *normal*.

**What you'll be tempted to do**

Know that you'll be tempted to shut it all out. You might be tempted to drink alcohol or do other things that help drown out the feelings and distract from the intrusive thoughts. You might be tempted to avoid work itself, to avoid the places and people that might trigger memories. You might be worrying that people at work are talking about the event or about you. Try to remember that these events will happen to all of us in our midwifery careers and that it's only when we talk that we feel the empathy of those around us. Empathy is much more likely than judgement. If or where there is judgement, it comes from a place of fear – that person is trying to remain safe, to avoid being the next person exposed to what you have just experienced. That doesn't necessarily help you in the moment, of course.

**What is best for your brain and your wellbeing**

For the next few days, eat well, exercise, try to sleep and rest when you can. Even when it's hard, try to talk about what happened, especially with those whom you trust. Get professional help from a trauma-informed service. Email for self-referral with the word 'trauma' or 'help' or 'incident' in the subject line. This means that you do not need to explain further. No text in the email is needed. The service is completely confidential and separate from both Trust HR and the maternity unit leadership. You can do this now if you want to. You may not think you need this, but if within 3–4 weeks you are still experiencing intrusive thoughts it is absolutely essential that you get this help for your brain to integrate what has happened in a healthy way.

## PSYCHOLOGICAL FIRST AID IS WHAT WE NEED

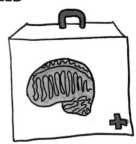

*Step 1: How we choose to see the intrusive thoughts*
The first step in psychological first aid is for all of us to understand and make friends with the sensations in our bodies.

Trauma memories are different from other types of memories. They are stored in the primitive fear centre of the brain and result in intrusive thoughts, dreams and memories, which are a difficult but entirely *normal* and rather clever attempt by the brain to try to trigger us to process and file them. They are like a messy wardrobe which, despite our best efforts to close the door, will keep bursting open, reminding us that it still needs sorting and tidying up.

Intrusions include a lot of sensory information and are often easily triggered, involuntarily, by stimuli associated with the event. Participants in Harvard Medical School's early fMRI studies in 1994 agreed to be re-triggered in the scanner with a co-agreed script of their traumatic event. The results show major activation of Brodmann's area 19 in the brain, an area in the visual cortex that registers images as soon as they enter the brain. Under normal circumstances these raw images would be quickly moved to other brain areas for interpretation, but here they show up as if the event is happening right now, in the present.[24] This can be devastating for those who have experienced trauma, as the brain makes us believe the threat is current, even in perfectly innocent moments, with a flashback triggered by a smell, a texture, a colour, a sound. In The BBC adaptation of *This is Going to Hurt*[25] we see Ben Whishaw playing the Adam Kay registrar character open the fridge at home and barely see the shape and texture of some kind of meat before it becomes a picture in his mind (still at the back of his fridge) of the 25-week-old baby he delivered the previous week after a devastating misdiagnosis. These visceral responses are normal, and you could even say helpful, hard though they are. They are evidence of our brain trying to facilitate our survival.

The other discovery using fMRI imaging also helps us to understand why the experience is so vivid and visceral: recalling trauma activates the right brain hemisphere while deactivating the left. Psychiatrist and trauma specialist Bessel van der Kolk describes the right hemisphere as carrying 'the music of experience'.[26] The first hemisphere to develop in the womb, it is used in non-verbal communication with our primary carer – body language, facial expressions, tone of voice – and goes on to store memories of smell, sound, touch and associated emotions. In the midst of trauma, when we most need our left hemisphere to help sequence our experiences and put overwhelming sensations into words, it is offline. Scans show, for example, Broca's area, one of the brain's speech centres often affected in stroke patients, completely deactivated during flashbacks.[27] There are no words. The body and memory are, in a sense, frozen in the experience of trauma, hindering any attempt to make 'sense' of it.

### Step 2: How we choose to respond to the intrusive thoughts

Avoiding the thoughts themselves is the most common reaction: to block or numb or distract away from painful thoughts or memories. That is why in the immediate aftermath of an event we are prone to using alcohol or drugs to numb, destructive behaviour including in our relationships: anything to direct attention elsewhere. We might also avoid places or things that might trigger the memories, including work, or try to avoid talking about them.

So the memories stay where they are, in the primitive fear centre, stuck; less likely to be integrated, causing further hypervigilance or hyperarousal in us.

We might then make meaning about the ongoing nature of these debilitating intrusions – that we are not strong enough, or resilient enough; that there is something fundamentally wrong with us feeling this way, especially when, after all, it's 'so much worse' for the family involved. This self-criticism – and the guilt and confusion it creates – might make us even less likely to get the help we really need, including the support of our peers and that of trauma-focused professionals who can help sort the wardrobe so that everything is in its rightful place.

The amazing brain can heal well by getting help to:

- Manage the intrusions – by acknowledging them, labelling them, and allowing them to pass by.

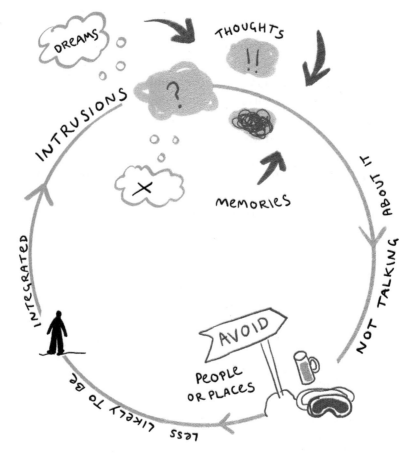

- Understand and empathise with our natural responses – being compassionate rather than critical with ourselves.
- Avoid the avoidance – recognising our unhelpful patterns and mitigating them.
- Reduce our isolation – by being in places, even with our peers, and also with trauma-informed professionals, where we can process experiences safely with no risk or judgement.[28]

Affected by a recent traumatic incident myself at work, I was lucky enough to be exposed to human kindness, and strong leadership in post-traumatic event response. I was also exposed to systems which, although not in any way perfect, were working: I was contacted by my Professional Midwifery Advocate (PMA) the next day to see if I needed any follow-up. Not everyone is this fortunate. On another day of the week, I might not have been so fortunate. Of the midwives in the 2021 study who needed psychological support after a traumatic event, all said that they did not feel prepared for the experience, that most traumatic births were largely ignored in their workplace, and that midwives received support mostly from their colleagues – risking of course inadvertent secondary traumatic stress in the listener.[29] An as yet unpublished 2023 joint RCM/RCOG good practice paper is seeking to support a culture change which is sorely needed around traumatic events and the handling of PTSD.[30]

The POPPY programme (Programme for the Prevention of PTSD in Midwifery) seeks to create a trauma-aware maternity workforce – with a workshop for all staff, information leaflet, peer support system, easy access to confidential rapid psychological support including a simple self-referral system, plus clear guidance for managers about handling investigations after traumatic events in a trauma-informed way. There is evidence that the programme reduces levels of PTS symptoms, decreases absence and increases satisfaction. Also, all those who accessed the rapid psychological support moved from clinical to non-clinical levels of PTSD.[31] There is a clear business case. The cost of having a functioning programme is less than £2 per week per midwife. So why aren't we all using this? One Trust in Liverpool is currently implementing POPPY. There was talk of it being included in the Royal College of Midwives' 'Caring for You' refresh in 2022, but even the mention of midwives' psychological trauma appears to be noticeably absent.

There have been some recent positive shifts in national policy. A psychological training 'boost' was made available nationally to PMAs in England in 2021-23, intended for PMAs to:

- Understand some common mental health disorders.
- Understand what trauma looks like.
- Learn techniques that the PMAs can implement with staff to help them manage emotions, and develop their own coping mechanisms.
- Learn ways that PMAs can manage their own wellbeing when potentially hearing more traumatic experiences than usual.[32]

This is good news – and it is evidently vital that in midwifery education and practice we engage with comprehensive awareness campaigns and action to create trauma-informed, compassionate, relational environments for families and midwives alike.

## A WORD ON POST-TRAUMATIC GROWTH

Post-traumatic growth focuses us (with strong, appropriate support) on the enquiry

'If something good was to come out of this, what might that be?'

Many of you will have heard of the Japanese art of *kintsugi*, literally 'joining with gold'. When a piece of pottery gets broken, it is mended lovingly by a craftsperson with molten precious metal, making the visible 'scars' part of its renewed beauty and now greater value. Trauma experience as midwives forms dramatic cracks in our sense of self and feelings about the world. With skilled, tender hands putting us back together, we, like the *kintsugi* bowl, can display some of our own healed scars. We may even be able to begin to see our own vulnerability as a gift rather than a liability,[33] capable of deepening our relationships and increasing our courage to speak out about what's important to us.

There are echoes of *kintsugi* in post-traumatic growth. Simply being aware of the idea of post-traumatic growth can be helpful: the knowledge that as a result of experiencing, then processing trauma, we as midwives might experience our own strength, make personal or professional decisions from a place of greater possibility, deepen our connection with others, appreciate life in a new way, even experience spiritual growth.[34-37] Positive growth after trauma can – given good support from the start – reduce fear and improve confidence and assertiveness[38,39] and reduce the risk of PTS in the future.[40,41]

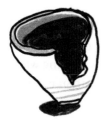 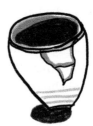

## RACISM AND OPPRESSION PUT BLACK AND BROWN MIDWIVES AT GREATER RISK OF TRAUMATIC STRESS

Systemic and interpersonal racism, health inequalities and disproportionality undoubtedly contribute to traumatic stress and moral injury among Black, Brown and Mixed Ethnicity midwives.[42]

The 2022 Birthrights report *Systemic Racism, Not Broken Bodies: An inquiry into racial injustice and human rights in UK maternity care*[43] gives vital context:

> 'In understanding systemic racism in healthcare, it is critical to appreciate the long history of dehumanisation of Black and Brown people in the UK. Throughout modern history, Black and Brown people have been perceived by white societies as being sub-human and Black women especially were subject to particular forms of abuse in healthcare settings, such as medical experimentation without consent and forced sterilisation. The medical model that exists in maternity care today was built on this patriarchal, white-supremacist framework.
>
> The echoes of this structure continue to exist in the treatment of Black and Brown people outside the parameters of 'normal', as normal is based on whiteness as the standard. This has an ongoing impact on many aspects of Black and Brown peoples' lives, including access to and provision of healthcare. The evidence in our inquiry illustrates that systemic racism and dehumanisation exists in maternity care in ways which threaten basic human rights to safety, dignity, autonomy and equality.'[44]

Black, Brown and Mixed Ethnicity recipients – and givers – of maternity care experience 'weathering': the lifetime impact of everyday racial trauma and discrimination on health[45] and its impact on the dynamics of trust.

Racial inequities in birth outcomes and experiences in the UK persist. We know that Black, Asian and Mixed Ethnicity women are respectively 3.7 times, 1.8 times and 1.3 times more likely to die in the perinatal period than White women.[46] Stillbirth rates of babies of Black and Black British families are over twice those for White babies and neonatal mortality rates 43% higher. For babies of Asian and Asian British ethnicity, stillbirth and neonatal mortality rates are both around 60% higher than for White babies.[47] Black women are up to twice as likely to have a severe pregnancy complication compared with White women.[48] The multi-layered explanation for these stark disparities clearly includes the impact of racism in the form of conscious and unconscious racial bias from healthcare professionals[49,50] shaping harmful attitudes, knowledge and assumptions.[51]

Dionne, a gentle, compassionate newly qualified midwife with a counselling qualification, and first-ever Black academic mentor at her university, told me her story:

> 'I've had years of being ignored in healthcare with my own health issues... I've been basically used as an experiment throughout my childhood with a skin condition. And after years of pain and being told in my mid-twenties that the only solution for my large fibroids was to have a hysterectomy, I finally found a team who listened to me.'

She describes looking after a Black woman in labour, and witnessing:

> 'judgement because of a part of her history, the "talk" outside the room, the looks, the rolling of the eyes, the body language changing. To be honest, I've always tried to block it out and just keep going.
>
> Black midwives and student midwives get upset or angry about being exposed to racism or triggering events, but it's the same thing we've had all our lives... these things happen, but there actually isn't anywhere you can go that is a safe space to talk about it, and for people to understand it and get it due to the lack of representation. So you just bury it. Then once it happens again, it comes up. That's very dangerous. I'm grateful that I'm so in tune – and I do things like journalling, five mins of meditation... and walking home to make space... because it can be a lot really... it can be monumental sometimes. There isn't really a safe space to speak to anybody. There are PMAs and all these wellbeing services, but if you were to voice what really happened,

*I don't think they'd take much notice. …you just become a bit of a troublemaker I suppose. You would get a label…'*

Dionne has also witnessed Black midwives themselves tuning out, and conforming to the prevailing culture:

*'As much as they want to be there and are there for those women, they just block it out. That really breaks my heart, when you see a Black midwife looking after a Black woman and they've adopted that negative attitude – it's just become a culture.'*

Dionne found a mentor among the university lecturers who became an inspiration and got her through. In practice, she struggled.

*'The majority of Black midwives at a central London teaching hospital who were actively nurturing the students and campaigning for change after the BLM movement in 2020 have left because they didn't feel heard and seen, even though they were involved in channels of communication between Black and Asian midwives and senior leadership.'* [52]

The NHS Workforce Race Equality Standard report[53] reveals the disproportionately low numbers of Black, Brown and Mixed Ethnicity midwives at Band 7 and above. These groups of midwives and maternity support workers (MSWs) are more likely than white midwives to experience bullying, harassment and discrimination at work, and more likely to face disciplinary proceedings,[54] and suspension (19.6% vs 6.3%) or dismissal (13.2% vs 0.7%) during disciplinary proceedings. The NHS staff survey 2021 reports 19.2% of Black, Brown and Mixed Ethnicity staff experiencing discrimination from service users or members of the public in the last 12 months (up from 16.7% in 2017). 17% said they had experienced discrimination from managers or colleagues in the last 12 months (up from 14.5% in 2019).[55] In the NHS *Turning the Tide* maternity report, in the wake of clear health disparities through Covid-19, 64% of staff respondents said that racism is ongoing and is rife in UK healthcare.[56]

Given newly qualified midwife Dionne's history as a Black woman who has directly experienced healthcare inequalities and discrimination, her cry is particularly searing. It echoes in many ways the voices of the women and families sharing their lived maternity experience as part of the Birthrights inquiry. As she says:

*'I need you to know me, and understand my situation to understand how I go about things. It's hard enough being with different mentors… it feels like the care element has been taken out when it comes to being a midwife or a mentor, the care element has gone… you're just left. Even the simple things… it just feels very lonely.'*

This is not to say, of course, that midwives and student midwives of every ethnicity and background might not share this cry. Yet how many more layers of trauma (historical and daily) are Black, Brown and Mixed Ethnicity colleagues dealing with? How much more care and attention is required when we finally wake up to our colleagues as individuals, and the collective harm they carry?[57] How much more can we ask, and truly listen to experiences (without burdening colleagues with the need to educate)? And as White majority midwives and leaders, how much more can we challenge each other on our implicit bias or explicit racist language or actions? How can we make this question visible and part of the 'daily checks': how is racism at work here? The Capital Midwife anti-racism framework being piloted across London could be a way into making these vital conversations more explicit.[58] Calling on the NMC to embed cultural safety into midwifery curricula, registration and revalidation, as it is in New Zealand, is another urgent next step.

Dionne's experience is echoed in the small 2021 survey run by the Association of South Asian Midwives CIC (ASAM) & Society of African & Caribbean Midwives (SoAC). Many of the 60 midwives attending an accompanying workshop had 'never had the courage to voice the type of racism and microaggressions they experience within the workplace'.[59]

*'When questioned about why there was a need to keep silent and tolerate the ongoing bombardment of negative behaviours, it was*

*apparent that the midwives believed that by raising these concerns it would be like throwing away one's career and that they would be labelled as being difficult and would have even more problems within the workplace. It was also mentioned that there are a large number of people that believe that racism does not exist and that the "race card" is used as a tool when things get tough or difficult.'*[60]

The mocking tone of a recent *Times* article (and accompanying assenting comments) about tackling micro-aggressions in the NHS suggests this kind of denial is alive and kicking.[61]

We are desperately in need of more large-scale and high-quality research in the area of the inequalities impacting mental health in Black and Brown and Mixed Ethnicity midwives and student midwives. We know for example from the 2020 Society of Occupational Health report on nursing and midwifery that only two of the many studies they analysed actually looked at ethnic differences in levels of wellbeing. Even in these two studies, however, the sample did not reflect the diversity of the nursing and midwifery population. The report revealed how sparse data on ethnicity is in research, and that if it is collected, it is not always clearly presented, making it difficult to see how representative samples actually are of diverse populations.[62]

From what we know of healthcare professionals in other specialities, Black, Brown and Mixed Ethnicity midwives may have additional vulnerabilities to trauma due to:

- Exposure to the same discrimination and racism as families in the maternity or health system.
- Possible close identification with clients of a similar background or with similar experiences, again influenced by being a recipient of discriminatory or racist behaviour in healthcare settings.
- Caseloads that might include more vulnerable or marginalised communities and/or extra interpreting or 'explaining' responsibilities such as contributing expertise about race and marginalised identities.
- Lack of baseline psychological or cultural safety in their place of work as experienced in ongoing micro-aggressions and discriminatory practices.

As Toni Morrison said in a panel conversation at Portland State University in 1975, 'the very serious function of racism' is distraction. 'It keeps you from doing your work. It keeps you explaining, over and over again, your reason for being'.[63]

Not only are Black, Brown and Mixed Ethnicity midwives experiencing systemic and structural racism[64] which is largely culturally denied, but the additional impact of trauma exposure in the workplace is also being denied or unacknowledged.

It's hard to deny, given recent news coverage in response to the Ockenden report[65] and the East Kent Maternity Services report,[66] that there are some major cracks in the foundations of maternity services. But even post-Ockenden in the NHS, social media posts and corporate communications at odds with reality persist, their images or words conveying the message:

*'Nothing wrong here.'*

*'Best job in the world...'*

This is extreme gaslighting. It denies the lived experience of all maternity staff, and it denies the experience of marginalised colleagues all the more harmfully.

## WHAT ABOUT OUR LEADERS? SENIORITY AND EXPERIENCE DON'T PROTECT

Surprisingly, perhaps, studies show a significant positive correlation between seniority and symptoms of PTSI and burnout. Even though years of experience might create a growing sense of competence and perhaps the ability to weather circumstances,[67,68] it very likely means increased exposure to potentially traumatic events.[69] This does not mean that it is the accumulation of traumatic events that may eventually affect the severity of PTSI symptoms; instead, it seems that more years in the job just mean a midwife is more likely to experience an event that is subjectively more traumatic.[70] All the more reason, it seems, to build robust processes with access to psychological support which has pathways independent of the direct colleagues around us. The hierarchical nature of the NHS maternity system also means that senior leaders report having fewer and fewer people to confide in, and the toxic combination of an enormous sense of responsibility for staff wellbeing and meagre tools or resources to meet the need. One senior leader told me that through two difficult years of peak Covid no one had asked her 'How are you?'. Until she had paused and reflected, she just hadn't noticed the absence of the question from others. Nor had she noticed that she hadn't asked the question of herself.

## WHAT ABOUT OUR STUDENTS – TRAUMA EXPOSURE FROM THE OUTSET?

*'Keep it inside, move on to the next lady cos you can't have what happened impact on somebody else but... if you do that and you keep everything inside and hold it all for yourself and try and deal with it all yourself, it's not a healthy way of being cos if you cannot unravel that... then it is just going to stay there. Because it is going to be like a ball of mess that you cannot undo.'* Student midwife[71]

Student midwives can of course also develop a trauma exposure response or post-traumatic stress symptoms as a result of witnessing traumatic births – either from a single episode or over time.[72] Studies of student midwives' exposure to traumatic events highlight feelings of vulnerability in the clinical environment. They reiterate the need to understand that any definition of 'traumatic' lies with the person involved, and reinforce what a difference supportive cultures would mean to students, making sense of experiences and growing self-awareness to aid resilience in the future.[73] How could we partner with our local universities to collaboratively show students 'the map' and encourage them to name and reflect on their experiences of occupational hazards and doubts about the future?

Educators, Clinical Placement Facilitators (CPFs) or equivalent, and practice supervisors can help in the following ways to support the emergence of self-aware and trauma-aware future midwives, who can go on facing unexpected events in practice.[74]

- Focusing on the inherent psychological complexities – making sure this is known and talked about as part of the role.[75] Making sure that while these complexities are 'normalised' they are also regarded as intense, challenging and a genuine hazard of the work.
- Discussing the neuroscience of trauma and the brain, both formally and informally, including implementing proactive interventions like the POPPY programme for students.[76]
- Addressing cultural safety, awareness, implicit bias and racism directly as a part of a decolonised midwifery curriculum that spirals through every aspect of learning and reflection. This is certainly beginning to happen in some UK universities. Then involve midwifery educators in supporting practice environments by opening up these conversations around trauma, racism and cultural safety.
- Creating safe, supportive, non-judgemental spaces to discuss stressful experiences, where a student's own perception of the event can be validated, and trauma processing in the brain can be supported.[77] There is some evidence suggesting that classical 'debriefing' (including critical incident debriefing) is actively unhelpful for trauma-exposed individuals, as it can reinforce the template of trauma in the brain.[78] But the importance of supported reflection time cannot be overestimated in developing awareness of the emotional dimensions of midwifery work and a deep, flexible future resilience.[79]
- Offering further support or therapeutic help where needed.[80]
- Establishing trauma-informed teams of 'Link Lecturers' specifically for Black, Brown and Mixed Ethnicity students, responsible for their wellbeing across the university placements spectrum.[81]

Davies and Coldridge, in their study of students' response to traumatic events,[82] use this powerful word to describe the midwife mentor or educator: a 'container'. They draw the comparison between the work we do for birthing women and families and the work we need to do for each other, even in the context of deeply challenging events.

> 'As [legendary midwife Tricia] Anderson noted, the role of the midwife in labour is to help women feel "safe enough to let go"; to

*provide a sense of security that enables women to safely enter the disconnected state and thus facilitate the birth process. Similarly educators and mentors/supervisors (all of us!) require a feeling language to contain the vulnerable student during the transition to midwife.'* [83]

If that isn't emotion work, I don't know what is!

And what if midwives themselves felt 'safe enough to let go' in order to facilitate that same containment for women and families?

## QUESTIONS FOR YOU: PTSI AND THE BRAIN

- What if anything feels like a relief as you read this chapter?
- Where do you feel seen?
- What will you do or say differently now?

# CHAPTER 9

# PSYCHOLOGICALLY SAFE ENVIRONMENTS, COMPASSIONATE LEADERSHIP AND INCIDENT HANDLING

Let's face it, the unexpected happens in maternity care. This adds to the need for psychological safety at work, which can not only mitigate the impact of traumatic events, but also prevent avoidable errors happening in the first place.[1] The Ockenden report comments specifically about the lack of psychological safety when a culture of 'them and us' is allowed to develop between obstetric and midwifery staff.[2] So how do we reset our culture, and what could a psychologically safe maternity ward/team look and feel like?

## THE STRONGEST FOUNDATION FOR PSYCHOLOGICAL SAFETY: VULNERABILITY

If you have heard of the work of Brené Brown, researcher on shame and vulnerability, you will understand the basic premise on which Resets 1, 2, and 3 are standing:

- Vulnerability is not weakness. That myth is profoundly dangerous, yet still pervasive in the battle-through coping culture[4] we have seeded, watered and grown in midwifery.
- Vulnerability involves emotional risk, exposure, uncertainty and it is our most accurate measurement of courage.

## RESETS FOR A PSYCHOLOGICALLY SAFE MATERNITY TEAM

### Expectation Reset 1

'staff should expect to work in a psychologically safe environment that can "hold" them when facing work-related challenges, rather than feel lucky if they happen to work in such a team/department.'[3]

### Expectation Reset 2

Expect that things will go wrong in ever-changing environments heavily influenced by human factors. Talk about this as a department regularly. Treat it as a 'when' not 'if' scenario. Open up multi-disciplinary discussion forums to hear from others. Rename the risk department 'team learning' or something that reflects the impossibility of perfect care and decision-making. Co-create organisational safety by welcoming those involved in adverse incidents (when appropriate) to help explore systemic change that might have made a difference. Create opportunities for leaders to share fears, regrets, vulnerabilities. Ironically, sharing fears and experiences is often seen as a 'risk' in itself: what if it were to open a Pandora's box of mental mess, including overwhelming fear and trauma? The reality is that mistakes thrive in silence, and guilt and shame thrive in the dark. Brought out into the light, they lose their power, which leaves more mental energy for caring for women and families and more straightforward, authentic relationships between staff.

### Expectation Reset 3

Expect and accept emotional challenge as a daily part of the work of a midwife and expect that staff will need ongoing emotional support and re-resourcing throughout their lives as midwives. Create opportunities for leaders to share publicly their own mental health journeys. Restructure the day, even very slightly, to enable handovers that include acknowledgement of challenges and successes, of human lives, feelings and needs.

- Vulnerability is the birthplace of connection. It is also the birthplace of creativity, innovation and change.[5]

The truth is, we're desperate for it – to witness vulnerability in others, and for the freedom or permission to be vulnerable ourselves. It connects us with others and takes away the loneliness of 'it's just me'.

And yet vulnerability is only possible in a psychologically safe environment. Vulnerability needs to be matched with the belief that we will be listened to, non-judgementally, by someone who ultimately has our back. Only then can we dare to bring our full selves to the situation and be vulnerable with people around us.

Fundamental to how the brain processes information is its obsession around safety and threat. At any moment the brain is taking in billions of data bits (most of which we are unaware of), pattern-matching them with what we have already encoded in our brains, in a bid to work out whether we are, in that moment, 'safe' or about to face a 'threat'. From an evolutionary perspective this has successfully kept us in the gene pool. In our modern world, it's not just sabre tooth tigers that can trigger a threat response: anything that undermines our sense of connectedness, our financial or physical security (think Maslow's hierarchy of needs again), or stokes our fears arounds failure, overwhelm or sense of self-worth, can activate the same series of chemical reactions that we experience as the racing heart and sweaty palms known as the 'fight, flight or freeze' response. The threat response is useful in that the adrenaline and cortisol give us heightened focus on the problem itself, and can elevate energy levels for a short period of time. The downside is that it switches off up to 40% of our cognitive capacity, hence our capacity to problem-solve, remember details or think outside the box can be impeded. And excessive activation of this threat response, as we've seen, can lead to burnout.

When the threat circuits activate, we narrow our focus (there are visual experiments that demonstrate how literal this is), and we can become problem-saturated, err on the side of pessimism and avoid or withdraw from tasks or other people.

One of the best ways to switch off this frequently activated 'homeland security system' is through a sense of connection with others. Oxytocin is an antidote to the adrenaline/cortisol mix. It is also longer lasting than a dopamine hit we get from alcohol, gambling, pressing save and send on that report, or anything else that we use to give us an artificial high to offset the feelings that come with the threat response (see the exercise on emotional regulation in Part II p.166)

In social groups, the extent to which we regulate or dysregulate each other is very fast-acting (pre-conscious even, as we are so sensitive to picking up emotions in others), so everyone has a role to play in this. Engaging with others who nourish us helps with self-regulation and when this is part of team culture it creates conditions for co-regulation, whereby we help each other manage our reactions to adverse situations. Supportive, collaborative, collegiate teams and departments become an antidote to threat and act as a buffer against worry and rumination.[6] Creating a culture of 'checking in', where we can ask 'how are you?' and have space to reply honestly, puts the person before the task and is the first step to vulnerability.

## THE LEADER AND TEAM IN RELATIONSHIP

Amy Edmondson uses her research[7] to invite us to respond to the following statements to determine the psychological safety of the teams we work in:

1. If you make a mistake on this team, it is often held against you -
2. Members of this team are able to bring up problems and tough issues +
3. People on this team sometimes reject others for being different -
4. It is safe to take a risk on this team +
5. It is difficult to ask other members of this team for help -
6. No one on this team would deliberately act in a way that undermines my efforts +
7. Working with members of this team, my unique skills and talents are valued and utilised +

Yes responses to the statements marked with a + and no responses to those marked with a - indicate that we are working in a team which feels psychologically safe. If the opposite is true, keep reading.

## SETTING UP PSYCHOLOGICAL SAFETY AT THE BEGINNING OF THE SHIFT

It's so tempting to 'just get on with the job'. That feeling is familiar to all of us. Especially when you have midwives around you waiting to get out of the door after a 12-hour shift, trying to catch a departing train or minimise the impact of school-run traffic. And yet the following tiny things go a long way to establishing a sense of psychological safety, especially in a rotating new-configuration-every-day team: warmth, a welcome, introductions – especially of new people, small celebrations, a leader indicating clear intentions: 'My job today is to provide you with the psychological safety you need: to enable you to feel well fed, watered, rested and trusted enough to be able to raise questions or concerns, to admit without fear the inevitable mistakes that are part of life and this work and to ask for what you need.' Adding a pinch of genuine vulnerability might add depth to the atmosphere and encourage staff to be more open and vulnerable themselves, e.g. 'I'm feeling a bit sad tonight because my mum's not well. It's likely that some of you are bringing things with you this evening, especially if you didn't sleep well'.

How different would you feel if a shift started like that? I would probably cry with relief. And of course I'm picturing the labour ward board with the stress of the whole unit weighing it down, but this could be just as applicable to a Band 6 leader on a postnatal ward working alongside a NQM with slight adaptations: 'Our job today is to give each other the psychological safety we need to do our jobs well and to ask for what we need from the doctors and the unit lead. What's going to make a difference to you today?'

This is a form of holding and presence both ways: a gentle emotional holding of another person in that moment which makes space and (even fractional) time for emotions, concerns or needs to arise and therefore to become more manageable.

If there is space/time for them, then they become warranted and justified.

And it is, as we know, largely absent from handovers as the focus remains on the board or handover sheet of people-to-be-processed, rather than the vital relationships with the team about to begin the work. It's a moment full of potential; a moment of 'being' among all the doing, and a mark of person-centred leadership.[8,9] Brief though it might be, it leaves us with a feeling of 'My cup is filled. I have capacity to pour out to you (other team member, woman or family).'

I am in no way underestimating what it takes to make space for even the smallest amount of connection or reflection in an action-orientated reactive environment, with action-orientated people. A 2020 pre-COVID study, looking at the impact of 'Recognise and Reflect' team sessions at the end of each weekday day shift, acknowledged the value of the sessions and yet discontinued 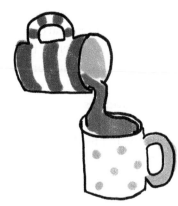 them anyway after five weeks as impractical.[10] Reflection is important. We know it, but we don't do it, or just can't find a way. Or maybe we offer it, but staff don't come, pressed as we are by the relentlessness of our day, or desperate as we are to get some mental space from work on our days off. Evidence is strong for the effectiveness of one-hour sessions like Schwartz Rounds, facilitated time to reflect on the ethical, emotional and social challenges at work around a big theme, to reduce psychological distress, normalise emotional responses to the intensity of health work and enhance ability to see differing perspectives. Immensely valuable as they are, Schwartz Rounds, reflective sessions, restorative clinical supervision and tea with the PMA are time 'out', rather than time 'in' our regular day.

The handover moment above is a micro 'time in' moment. What other moments can you picture in a clinical day when psychological safety might be reinforced? What might the end of the day look like?

## WE ARE ALL LEADERS

We can all take responsibility for this and play our part. We are all leaders in our own lives and in our spheres of influence (see p.121 for a helpful question for all of us to pose for ourselves; see p.216

in Part II for an exercise on our sphere of control and sphere of influence). And it is certainly true that those midwives who are leaders in the hierarchy have a particular burden and joy of creating and maintaining psychological safety. Pam Smith's seminal work on emotional labour and psychological safety in nursing emphasised how the ward leader clearly sets the emotional tone for students, who were able to care *only* when they were being cared for.[11]

Karen Ledger, in her chapter in Jan Smith's *Nurturing Maternity Staff*, calls on leaders to ask some great questions which can enhance self-awareness in this area:

- Why do I lead? (i.e. what's the purpose of the leading that I do; what am I trying to shape or create?)
  and
- Who do I want to *be* as a leader?[12]

Any one of us can answer these questions and find it helpful, no matter where we are in our midwifery journey. This absolutely includes student midwives, directors of midwifery and everyone in between. And the leaders in the hierarchy are lost without the clear sense of purpose and direction these questions produce.

Sheena Byrom's awakening about compassionate, relationship-based leadership, as described in *Nurturing Maternity Staff*, brings so much wisdom. She recalls as a midwifery manager feeling distant from the care and connection she once offered to women and families. She noticed that bringing the same level of awareness, presence and kindness to her staff members could bring deep satisfaction, increased safety and positive outcomes all round.[13] She used her well-honed midwifery skills to connect more deeply with staff.

Listen to the echoes of midwifery practice in Brené Brown's description of empathy: 'we can respond empathically only if we are willing to be present to someone's pain',[14] and 'We need to dispel the myth that empathy is "walking in someone else's shoes". Rather than walking in your shoes, I need to learn to listen to the story you tell about what it's like in your shoes *and* believe you even when it doesn't match my experiences.'[15] (My emphasis.)

A person-centred, compassionate leader fosters a culture of trust and belonging, and creates a highway of accessibility for someone like Amity Reed in the midst of burnout:

> 'If I'd felt confident that my work-inflicted mental health problems would've been taken seriously by my employers, that I would've received non-judgemental support and given enough time and tools to heal, I'd have reported my concerns and sought help much earlier. The NHS is not currently set up to support staff at an individualised level and is often shrouded in fear and defensive practice, which contributes massively to people being too frightened of losing their careers or reputations to come forward. This needs to change to prevent experiences like mine from becoming more commonplace.'[16]

The evidence for relational leadership is strong. A 2018 analysis of 129 research studies in nursing showed that leadership based on task completion rather than relationship leads to lower productivity, job satisfaction and retention of staff.[17] Relationship-based leadership also grows a culture of belonging rather than 'fitting in', where as an individual I can see that I am wanted, I am valued, I can contribute more than the basic functionality of my role – a vital element of all diversity, equity and inclusion work. A culture of belonging requires vulnerability, and the discomfort of figuring out how to be alongside people and have meaningful conversations without letting go of who we are or what's important to us. 'Fitting in' is being accepted for

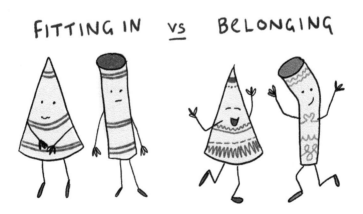

FITTING IN vs BELONGING

being just like everyone else: just as efficient, just as cynical, just as hilarious, just as war-weary. Brené Brown describes fitting in as a 'threat' to a culture of belonging.[18]

The 'shadow' the leader casts is really important – their influence on those around whether present or not.[19] Team members have a long, clear memory for feelings of lack of psychological safety.[20] The leader is always modelling (consciously or not) 'how we behave around here', always being observed for how words line up with actions, and always has the potential to model a culture of belonging and the vulnerability that feeds it, especially if it's also being modelled from the top of the organisation or department. Obstetrician and voice of 'human factors' in maternity Ruth-Anna talks in *Nurturing Maternity Staff* about her own involvement in a tragedy, and the life-changing impact of colleagues finally telling her their own vulnerable stories of errors, failures and learning. She says:

> 'it was one of the most important contributors to me still being in the speciality and able to see a future for myself in obstetrics. It's absolutely not easy. Egos are fragile, medicine is famously hierarchical and in many ways it functions due to a belief that doctors... are infallible. This erroneous belief not only damages individuals, who feel they are alone in their distress, but is also a huge factor in missed institutional learning.'[21]

Shame and guilt – and repeat patterns of behaviour – thrive in the dark. Vulnerable moments cast a powerful light.

## TRUST

Compassionate and relational leadership in action seeds the core ingredient of a psychologically safe environment: trust. Charles Feltman, in *The Thin Book of Trust: an essential primer for building trust at work*, defines trust and distrust in the following striking way. As you read the descriptions, notice the people/teams/leaders you picture, or what happens in your body in response to the words. Try reading them twice.

**Trust**: *'choosing to risk making something I value vulnerable to another person's actions'. (That could be your reputation, your current family or health challenges, your name, your feelings in that moment, your history or ethnicity, your beliefs…)*
**Distrust**: *'what's important to me is not safe with this person in this situation (or any situation)'.*[22]

Every one of us knows the feeling of navigating trust and distrust in ever-changing teams and in high-stress, high-stakes environments; that lingering question of 'Who has got my back?'

*'If the delivery suite co-ordinator was nice, participants felt positive within their work and level of morale. They knew who to ask if they were unsure what to do and definitely knew who to avoid.'*[23]

When an early career midwife says that she is 'too intimidated to ask for help due to attempts to humiliate myself and other newly qualified staff in front of colleagues by senior members of staff',[24] we can see a deep river of distrust because shame and humiliation have been used as a tool of power. There is no psychological safety, and the safety of the families in our care is simultaneously being sacrificed. As Elie Wiesel, holocaust survivor, human rights activist and Nobel peace prize winner, summarised his life's work:

*'Never allow anyone to be humiliated in your presence.'*

Feltman's commentary on his 4 Distinctions of Trust (below) is helpful here. He says that we are always making assessments of another person's trustworthiness. Of the four areas we are scanning, research shows that 'Care' is the most important for building lasting, deeper trust: the kind that makes us feel safe being vulnerable. We may be able to trust a colleague's sincerity, reliability and competence, but if we don't think they consider our humanity and interests, we may limit our trust to specific situations or transactions, rather than trusting that colleague more broadly. In other words, without the 'Care' of compassionate and relational leadership, we can only operate with a transactional day-to-day quasi-'effectiveness', which leaves the human soul adrift.

**Sincerity** – *is the assessment that you are honest, that you say what you mean and mean what you say; you can be believed and taken seriously. It also means when you express an opinion it is valid, useful, and is backed up by sound thinking and evidence. Finally, it means that your actions will align with your words.*
**Reliability** – *is the assessment that you meet the commitments you make, that you keep your promises.*
**Competence** – *is the assessment that you have the ability to do what you are doing or propose to do. In the workplace this usually means the other person believes you have the requisite capacity, skill, knowledge, and resources to do a particular task or job.*
**Care** – *is the assessment that you have the other person's interests in mind as well as your own when you make decisions and take actions.* [25]

## WHAT'S NEEDED AFTER AN 'INCIDENT'? THE ULTIMATE PSYCHOLOGICAL SAFETY MOMENT

There are daily incidents, big and small, in maternity. Some are major; some feel major in our internal worlds. Some are officially classified as serious incidents. Jan Smith in *Nurturing Maternity Staff* discusses the power and possibility of a healing rather than a harmful approach after a serious incident, when staff are especially vulnerable to feelings of shame and at risk of ostracising themselves or being ostracised as speculation abounds. She names the crucial elements of any post-incident moment, including shifting the focus from the shame and blame-provoking question 'Who did it?' to a more factual 'What happened?' [27] The choice of tone for 'What happened?' also seriously influences the consequences for the second victim. An authentically-held underlying assumption that no one intends to harm, and that mistakes happen, softens the tone and enables the midwife to reverberate with shock (or begin writing a statement) in an atmosphere without shame (see Expectation Reset 2 in the box at the beginning of this chapter). Indeed, given that in the immediate aftermath of an incident our sympathetic nervous system is in full flight, the most soothing and humane words/stance are not 'What happened?' but 'How are you right now?' or even 'No need to say anything. I'm just here with

## WE ARE ALL LEADERS – A WHAT IF MOMENT

Provocative as this might sound in a hierarchical culture, often reinforced with uniforms, badges and incremental titles, we are all leaders: required to 'lead' in a multitude of ways in our personal and professional lives, influencing and shaping the environments we have chosen. One of the reasons why this statement is so provocative is that a hierarchy in itself (along with other factors) can disempower the natural sense of leadership in all of us and feed a culture of resentment, a culture of them (the senior managers) and us (the ones who do the work). Brené Brown helps us to understand that this resentment grows in the muddy waters between expectations (often unexamined and unexpressed) and disappointment. She asks us another 'what if' question.

*What if, instead of looking at that person and saying what they are doing wrong or should be doing, I asked myself this question:*

*What do I need but am afraid to ask for?*

*(I need X but worry that if I ask I will look X, etc)*

What a phenomenally liberating question this is. It can free us from the shackles of 'it's just the way it is' and give us a sense of our own part in the dance. Move from external locus of control – it's all happening out there – to an internal one with greater autonomy and freedom to move.

Brené Brown notes from her research how often we choose to live disappointed – numbing, being cynical, critical or semi-engaged at best – rather than risk feeling disappointment if we were brave enough to work out what we need and then ask for it.[26]

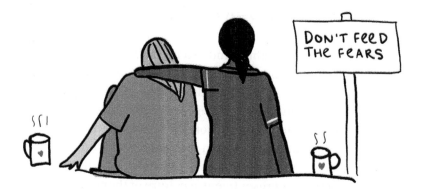

you.' (See p.93 for a response which soothes the autonomic nervous system immediately after an incident.)

The research shows that compassionate or relationship-based leadership makes an enormous difference to staff involved in adverse incidents.[28] A recent in-depth Norwegian study reflects something we have all experienced: how (as the authors describe it) an ad hoc, absent or untrustworthy style from a leader adds to feelings of guilt and shame in the second victim. A feeling of abandonment comes through strongly from many of the midwives in the study:

> 'I have thought many times that we do not have good follow-up routines after critical incidents. You feel abandoned, and you have no one to lean on.'[29]

> 'In retrospect, I feel the manager should have been there to support me. She never contacted me.'[30]

> 'Support after a critical incident depends on which colleagues you work with that day.'[31]

> 'We need a safe forum to share with our colleagues. If there is an adverse outcome, we are told to keep silent. There is no place to talk to unburden our souls.'[32]

By contrast, proactive rather than reactive responses mitigate the impact for the midwife: being visible and consistent as a leader, being present in and to the situation and all those affected, systematic routines in terms of post-incident response.

To the leader in this moment: when all else has melted away – and the midwife is imagining this to be a watershed moment in her career – she needs to know that she is fundamentally of value.

## AFTER AN INCIDENT: MOVING FROM A PLACE OF DISGRACE TO A PLACE OF GRACE

**What if** it could look like this?

### In the room
A room is dedicated to post-incident support (not the bereavement suite with its own triggers or any-old-office-just-because it's there. The investment in space and the right people is part of what signals how important this is).
The person receives a warm drink and emotional first aid – a reassuring presence first and foremost, then words with a tone focused solely on allowing the activated nervous system to regulate, possibly via normal physiological responses of trembling or shaking. (See p.93).
What happened is acknowledged without blame or judgement. Space is given for the person to experience all the responses in their body and any feelings present.
Clear signposting happens to easily accessed, fully confidential pathways for further support – preferably by self-referral.
The person is connected to a channel of information about the family's wellbeing.

### When the person is ready (possibly on another day)
A reflective discussion might happen about the details of the incident, with support and time offered to write any statement needed.
The person is given opportunities to meet with the family for a substantive conversation where appropriate.[33]

> ### When the person is ready (possibly on another day)
> Other people involved in the incident might also be invited (in paid time) to an opportunity to reflect as a group, and begin to contribute vital learning for the organisation. The focus remains:
> * We expect these things to happen…
> * How are you now?
> * What can we learn together?
>
> ### Outside the room
> A culture of strict honour and confidentiality around the event is maintained by leaders to minimise speculation and corridor talk. Because mandatory training includes trauma-informed post-incident practice and everyone knows 'the worst is over' scripts (see p.93), there is less fear in the air anyway, and less need for speculation or separation.

It's easier to write that list than to put it into practice. There are two layers here: putting into place systematic routines of 'what we know will help', and also the timing and tone with which it is delivered. We know from research in this area that the timing of processes immediately after an adverse incident is often exquisitely poor – and can be actively harmful to those involved. We've known for some time that even psychological debriefing, usually regarded as a positive move, is not effective in preventing PTSD developing by three months after an incident and can instead do harm.[34] We also know how inhumane and harmful it can feel to midwives having to write a statement at the end of a long shift in the midst of a fresh experience of trauma.[35] Jan Smith, in *Nurturing Maternity Staff,* also highlights the missed opportunity of a healing moment where staff say a heartfelt sorry to the family involved. The fear of adding fuel to the fire of litigation means that this moment is often missed or avoided. Its very absence not only adds oxygen to the fire, but also takes away a crucial moment of humanity and honesty for all involved.[36] Jan leads workshops for maternity staff with a lawyer entitled, 'Saying Sorry Doesn't Mean Litigation…' in recognition that both sides usually want this, but that perceived or real organisational barriers can make it very difficult indeed.

*'You don't get any formal training. I don't remember at any point
in my training someone saying you're going to have something that
will happen to you in your career that will make you never want
to go back to work and will make you doubt your ability to do your
job properly [...] Because you prepare soldiers on the battlefield
for how they might feel when they get home. I'm not likening it to a
battlefield but it's still a traumatic event.'* Midwife 129[37]

An ongoing investigation is also a source of much anxiety for
maternity staff and can create spiralling mental health. Ruth-Anna,
obstetrician, quoted in *Nurturing Maternity Staff*, describes each
later stage of the investigation as like a metaphorical ripping off
of the plaster.[38] If the case involves litigation, we are exposed to an
unfamiliar, lengthy process coming from an adversarial rather than
relational place, which puts us at risk of prolonged psychological
harm.[39] Midwives report feeling like 'collateral damage' or faulty
goods, especially if they are still working where the incident
happened, and are crying out for confidential sources of support and
organisational cultures which still put their wellbeing at the heart of
an investigation process.[40]

There remains much to be done.
And there is hope.

Caroline Hollins Martin, Elaine Beaumont and their team are
researching the use of Compassionate Mind Training to help midwives
cope with traumatic clinical incidents, designed to balance the threat
drive and soothe systems, settle the nervous system and encourage
reflection.[41] See Part II for compassion-based methods that you can
use in practice.

Interesting research is coming out of the conflict in Ukraine
in terms of treating acute refugee mental health (especially
PTSI symptoms) efficiently. Emily Holmes, Professor of Clinical
Neuroscience at Uppsala University, is working on a systematic
three-part package using a Tetris-based computer game on a phone
(rather than resource intensive verbal therapy) to dampen down
vivid and distressing images, with the aim in the longer term of taking

away the intrusive nature of the memories.[42] Marit Sijbrandij of Vue University Amsterdam has been training peer refugees to offer brief psychological interventions (five sessions face-to-face or online) for Syrian refugees. They have had excellent results, with a clear improvement in daily functioning treating symptoms of depression and PTSI.[43] Trauma best practice is an example of where those of us in maternity could benefit enormously from raising our eyes beyond our immediate horizon, and collaborating globally (for example with a growing number of specialists via the online global International Trauma Consortium) to find creative alternatives to care for a beleaguered workforce.

## QUESTIONS FOR YOU: PSYCHOLOGICAL SAFETY AND COMPASSIONATE LEADERSHIP

- What are you discovering about the psychological safety/lack thereof in your environment?
- Who can you talk to about this?
- What tiny moves can you make personally to enhance the psychological safety of colleagues (think small is beautiful)?
- What has made the most difference to you post-incident? What do you need more of?

# CHAPTER 10

# RESILIENCE – REALLY?

*'Revolution not resilience'*. Amity Reed, battle cry of *Overdue: Birth, Burnout and a Blueprint for a Better NHS*

*'Toughen up? I've been a soft-hearted health professional for 34 years and I've managed to survive.'* Joy Horner, independent midwife

Resilience has become a buzz word, often lazily applied as a sting in the tail, a watchword for 'grin and bear it'. And partly through the intensity of the Covid crisis, it has become very mixed up with the mindfulness movement. Ron Purser, Professor of Management at San Francisco State University, has practised mindfulness for decades and understands the strong neuroscientific evidence base, but is actively challenging the way that mindfulness is being used.[1] In his book *McMindfulness*, he exposes how mindfulness, the biomedical paradigm it comes from (stress is an individual pathology), and the industry that surrounds it, has been co-opted as a way of helping us stay focused on ourselves rather than identify what needs to change in the system. In other words it might help us 'tolerate the intolerable'.[2] He highlights the distortion that stress is seen as a maladaptation of the individual to the environment. Purser believes that rather than being used in the way that it is most helpful, to raise collective consciousness of what needs to change, it has become a convenient technique or salve for the corporate (or NHS) world, which may be failing to look at the structural and systemic causes of stress. He cites the almost absurd vision of employees at the notoriously harsh Amazon distribution warehouses having a brief mindfulness stop mid-shift in their 'Ama-zen' coffin-like upright booths.[3]

The truth is, it all feels so complex that we have reached for the neatly packaged solution which asks the individual to look inside. This is, you could argue, the ultimate definition of gaslighting: if you keep telling people that *they* are the problem, eventually they will believe it, or stop looking outside themselves and seeing what's actually broken.

Again, none of this discussion is to deny the validity and power of mindfulness in and of itself, but the question lies in how it is directed. Mindfulness-based stress reduction (MBSR) training over eight weeks has a strong evidence base and features in multiple NICE guidelines as a valid and often transformational way of approaching clinical diagnoses.[4]

UK psychologist and maternity ally Jan Smith expresses her concerns that resilience training in NHS maternity departments is actually 'training staff to tolerate a deeply broken system.'[5] Billie Hunter and Lucie Warren, in their 2022 revisiting of the concept, acknowledge that the term 'resilience' has been 'misappropriated by organisational imperatives'[6] as a way to shift responsibility back to the individual rather than act on much-needed changes to conditions and ways of working.[7] Unsurprisingly, studies have found that individual so-called 'self-care' strategies are only moderately effective at reducing burnout, empathic strain and trauma exposure response compared to organisational changes offering improved conditions, more control over work patterns, quality supervision, reduced exposure to trauma and structured group meetings for support.[8] There is also evidence from resilience research that strong relationships with role models who support a healthy reframing of realities and foster a sense of meaning (the so-called shift and persist model), can enhance resilience, even in people with ACEs or other baseline vulnerabilities.[9] In midwifery this could be realised in the form of enduring 1–1 mentoring or even reverse-mentoring relationships with time dedicated to co-reflection and learning.

The truth is that resilience is not about dodging or 'bouncing back' from psychological distress, or about developing a thick skin, or adorning ourselves with imagined badges of honour for coping against the odds.[10] It's rather the opposite. Resilience involves developing enough self-awareness to notice when we are overwhelmed or overrun, and taking small compassionate actions that help shift us gradually back to a better mental space. Hunter and Warren's original work on self-reported 'resilient' midwives supports this. These midwives use 'protective self-management', drawing on self-awareness to recognise stress triggers or warning signs and take active steps to minimise their impact.[11]

So growing self-awareness is the first step, along with using strategies to support the body and mind. An essential part of true resilience is to seek out (and give) support at challenging moments, which may then help mobilise us with the courage to call out negative behaviours, or the features of a dysfunctional system. Part II of this book not only provides practical tools to develop the features of 'resilience', but also helps us rediscover our purpose and meaning in this work, an antidote to the protective disengaged stance often seen as an essential survival (or quasi-resilience!) strategy in the NHS.

Of course, what often gets in the way is the so-called psychological contract: the unspoken expectations, beliefs and obligations of the role as perceived by the employer and employee; not the legal contract, but the 'understood way of working' that in reality can be totally unacceptable but has become the norm.

Midwife Grace sheds light on this, reflecting on her choices after joining a continuity team:

> I chose me, in that I stopped agreeing to work when I was exhausted; I chose me, in that I took rest when I needed and sought help when I was struggling even if others tried to convince me I was fine (for the benefit of the service); I chose me, in that I made a conscious effort to celebrate and value success that could not be measured with numbers or status. That made all the difference between how I viewed myself, my career choices and my self-worth, making it easier to enjoy the seemingly "small" wins.' [12]

## QUESTIONS FOR YOU: RESILIENCE - REALLY?

- What messages have you received about 'resilience' during your career? How have they helped/hindered you?
- What unspoken 'ways of working' exist in your situation? In which ways are they helpful or unhelpful?
- How is this (re)shaping your view of yourself in your current workplace?

# CHAPTER 11

# WHEN MIDWIVES GIVE BIRTH

*'There is no greater agony than bearing an untold story inside you'.* Maya Angelou, *I Know Why The Caged Bird Sings*[1]

What about midwives who are mothers or fathers, and the impact of their own birth/early parenting experiences on their experience of others', or their ability to care for families and be with the ambiguity and emotions that accompany the perinatal period?

This is a great unanswered question.

A 2021 study attempted to explore it by reviewing the literature on midwives and birth trauma, and found zero relevant studies (of 352 articles reviewed) to include: zero – a total gap in the literature; a so-called 'empty review'.[2]

How can that be?

This situation can only be explained by two enormous disconnects in our thinking: firstly, a complete absence of focus on the emotional health of a largely female midwifery workforce, the majority of whom will experience the seismic transition of birth and early parenting during or before their time as a midwife; secondly, a profound unwillingness to link the emotional health of midwives (including their personal primary trauma) with the emotional health of women (with their personal primary trauma) and take either as seriously as they deserve.[3]

Midwives with previous birth trauma of their own appear to be predisposed to PTSI – a recent study suggests this group are 42% more likely to develop PTSI symptoms in their professional life.[4] As negative interpersonal interaction during a traumatic event appears to be the highest predictor of trauma among women (over and above the objective 'severity' of the events themselves), there will be plenty of triggers in the path of the midwife who has also given birth. Of the 943 participants in a recent study of people giving birth, 748 (79%) responded to the qualitative question 'describe the birth trauma and what you found traumatising'. 66.7% of those described care provider actions and interactions in the following categories as the most traumatising elements of their experience: 'prioritising the care provider's agenda'; 'disregarding embodied knowledge'; 'lies and threats' and 'violation'.[5] So you could argue that a midwife's own conflicted provision of care as well as challenging interpersonal interactions with colleagues could act as triggers for any unresolved personal birth trauma.

As a midwife, this starts to blow your mind.

## MIND-BLOWING THOUGHTS

Given that around 30% of childbearing women experience perinatal trauma,[6] at least 30% of midwives who have given birth are carrying an experience of trauma back into a workplace that could be triggering and therefore provide opportunities for further trauma exposure. We know that midwifery events perceived as traumatic sometimes hold personal significance for midwives, in some way chiming with their own life experience.[7]

A lack of research means we don't yet know whether a midwife is more or less likely to experience birth trauma herself than a non-midwife. My suspicion is that given the number of midwives reporting exposure to traumatic events – 93.7% in a recent Australian study[8] – we are primed for trauma.

Adding to this, Black, Asian and Mixed Ethnicity women are 3.7 times, 1.8 times and 1.3 times as likely compared with White women to die in the perinatal period,[9] twice to three times as likely to have a baby who dies in the womb or after birth,[10] and more likely to experience 'care' as traumatic as a result of previous experience of trauma and marginalisation in healthcare.[11] How are we also paying attention to the complex layers of feelings among these groups of colleagues? What can we do? (See p.213 for a small change, big impact possibility).

The reality is this: midwifery education is missing its crucial role to facilitate deep reflection on birth/parenthood for those who are already mothers or fathers before they enter training. And maternity systems are neglecting the rich opportunity not just for healing, but also for growth that could come from quality, supported reflection on our own experiences of birth, feeding journeys and early parenting as midwives, female and male alike. Without it, we end up carrying our unprocessed stories around with us and creating armour in the form of scripts which can lead to blind spots or less openness to others' experience. Reflecting well, and with good structures and support, allows us to integrate our own stories and see the scripts we have developed around them and move into a more conscious relationship with our lives and work.

## QUESTIONS FOR YOU: WHEN MIDWIVES GIVE BIRTH

For those who have given birth at the same time as being a midwife:
- What might have made a difference in your pregnancy in terms of processing your midwifery journey/trauma?
- What would 'thoroughly emotionally supported' have looked like on your return to work?
- What are you discovering about how your own pregnancy/birth has (re)shaped you as a midwife?

For those midwives who have not been pregnant/given birth (but may be planning it!):
- What extra support might you now choose to seek out in your own pregnancy/to prepare you for birth?
- Who can support you in designing a return to work which is compassionate and trauma-informed (think your peers as well as midwifery leaders)?
- How has this chapter (or the rest of Part I) raised your awareness of what you need for the road ahead?

# CHAPTER 12

# YOU, THE MOUNTAINS AND THE JOURNEY

Welcome to the end of Part I. We have acknowledged the tangled strands of the psychological impact of our work. We have given words and voice to the experiences of midwives, student midwives and others in maternity care. The mountains are more visible and prominent now. Yet some of us will feel that just because we can see them more clearly, the dangers of thin air and harsh terrain are no less overwhelming – because we're there right now. Others of us will find it helpful to be able to see the landscape, to recognise and label the places we have been, often through deeply challenging times, in the fog of dense clouds.

Through our careers, even over a single day, we are all climbing or descending the five mountains of midwifery – sometimes one at a time, sometimes feeling the impact of all of them, all at once. In better times, or on better days, we might be walking through the foothills, the air more oxygenated, the ground more lush. We might witness others experiencing 'peak' distress, struggling to breathe, and remember our journey on that mountain. We might step in to help, resourcing that colleague with this map for awareness, with the right boots, crampons and ropes to optimise safety, with snacks that actually nourish and sustain, and finally with a promise of time at basecamp together with time to really listen. Part II is full of resources just like these – ways for us to uncover what makes us tick, ways to move the breath, the body and the mind to support ourselves and each other. Wherever you are right now in your journey through the mountains, Part II is for you.

## A WORD ABOUT SEEKING PROFESSIONAL HELP

Some of you will have been stirred up by stories of colleagues in the midst of depression, anxiety, addiction and self-harm. Some of you will be living them, or using those strategies for survival. If that is you, please talk to your GP or, if it feels safe, your occupational health team at work. Sadly, and somewhat comfortingly, they will be expecting you. Tell a trusted friend at work and work out a small next step together. Please don't suffer alone.

## QUESTIONS FOR YOU: END OF PART I

- What are you angry about/stirred up about?
- What does that make you want to explore further – about yourself/ with others?
- What do you know now that you didn't know before reading this? (About yourself or about the emotional/psychological challenges of midwifery)
- Who do you need/want to talk to about this?

# PART II

# EXPERIMENTING WITH NEW WAYS OF BEING AND CHOOSING

# INTRODUCTION

To use a phrase much loved by Brené Brown, I am a mapmaker and a traveller. And so are you.

That is to say, we don't have all the answers.

What we have here is a map of the midwifery landscape, plotted out together in Part I of this book, on which you have hopefully been able to trace some of your journey, or spot the 'places' or 'experiences' you have visited or taken up residence. From the map as it stands you will already be able to answer the question 'Where am I now?'

Part II takes us to a more personal place of map-making and meaning-making. We get to ask and answer the questions:

- Who am I?
- How did I get from there to here?
- How do I get from here to there?

We can add to the map the personal contours of 'biology, biography, behaviour and backstory'[1] which will reinvigorate your sense of yourself and your purpose. We will then get really practical: creating practices and using language in the whole of life and work that will raise your awareness of what you're feeling and what you need. You then also have the choice to use your newly refined voice and purpose to adopt a 'small change, big impact' mini project with a tribe of like-minded souls to implement in your team/environment.

## HOW TO USE PART II

The reflections and exercises are designed to be small and simple, but they are not always easy. At the heart of each of them are coaching questions which go to the core of you – questions such as:

- Who am I becoming?
- What am I tolerating?
- What is it to be undaunted?
- What am I actively choosing this week?

Or, as Mary Oliver asks in her poem 'The Summer Day':

*'Tell me what is it you plan*
*To do with your one wild and precious life?'*

These questions require daring to even go near them; a willingness to be *vulnerable enough* to see what's here – and choose what you *really* want. You are showing that honest vulnerability by picking up this book in the first place. I acknowledge you for that.

## A FEW TIPS TO MAKE THE MOST OF THE JOURNEY

**Get a partner:** we all know that accountability works. Try working through the book and the exercises with a colleague with whom there is mutual respect and some knowledge of each others' stories. Design how you want to support each other and commit to the road ahead.

**Get a rhythm:** whether you are travelling solo or with a colleague, commit to a regular time each week to come back to the exercises. Just as with a physical challenge or injury, we sign up to the training or rehab needed to see a shift happen or get well again: this is the same. This is like rehab for the mind, and for the new muscles we are growing which support our stronger self.

**Get writing:** write in this book if you're reading it on paper. Note-take if it's on a device. Choose a journal/ book in which to capture your reflections and discoveries. It will become a rich repository of insights about you which, once known, can't be unknown. It will be full of your 'colour', your 'flavour', which will then go on serving you every time you apply for a new job, revalidate, choose a life partner, a new home and so on. Nothing is wasted.

**Get moving:** don't imagine you have to sit still to do this work. In fact, when the body moves, so does the mind. So go walking with the exercise in hand (or in ears). Respond as you walk. Record your responses or thoughts if you prefer onto a voice note or recording.

**Get free range:** doing the exercises in Chapter 13 first will benefit you. They are designed to help you recall a stripped back version of you, fully alive, with dreams and a sense of purpose. However, don't get stuck on anything. Try the next exercise, ask your colleague for help to clarify what you're thinking or scootch along to chapters 14 or 15.

**Get a coach:** a coach is a person trained to be deeply curious about what you want for your life, to walk alongside you and ask great questions as you discover the heart of who you are and who you want to be. A relationship with a coach is one of accountability, fun and exploration – and the work you do together profoundly changes the way you see yourself and how you show up in your life.

Please feel free to contact me @wildrubiescoach with comments or feedback

# CHAPTER 13

# FIRST PRINCIPLES: PASSION AND PURPOSE

*'Staying healthy in a system that undermines your very existence is the greatest act of resistance'.* Audre Lorde[1]

### 10 THINGS I APPRECIATE ABOUT MYSELF

It is not often that we notice, much less note down, what we appreciate about ourselves. Our picture of ourselves is often made up of fragments gleaned from the views and comments of others, or assumptions we have made along the way, leaving an image a little like a reflection in a cracked mirror: visible but not entirely aligned. This, and the exercises to follow, is designed to bring you a clearer and more nuanced picture of your distinctive qualities.

- Don't think too much about this one. Treat it as a playful exercise.
- Set a one minute timer and write down 10 things you like about yourself.
- If you haven't yet made it to 10, reset the timer for one more minute and keep going... try 'I like the way I...'; 'I'm...'; single words are okay too, but including the 'I' helps you claim it as yours.
- If you're finding this tricky, think 'what were the qualities I demonstrated at work/at home yesterday (even when it wasn't going well...)?' Flexibility, courage to speak up for someone, humour, focus, creativity, openness... When do people turn to you for help?
- Share what you have written with an accountability partner or small group. Notice what it's like to share this. Ask them not to respond right now: you'll get a chance to ask them later what they appreciate about you.

## ASKING AN IMPORTANT QUESTION TO FIVE PEOPLE IN MY LIFE

This involves some daring (and therefore some vulnerability) and is *so rewarding.*

How often in our lives do we actually ask others to give their impressions of us? In writing, ask five people (three whole life, two work life), the simple question 'Who am I to you?'

Don't act on the 'need' to explain. Use this template if it helps:

*Dear X, I'm currently working on some exercises/working with a small group exploring what makes me tick and my impact on others. I have chosen you as one of five people to respond to this question: 'Who am I to you?'*

*Please get back to me by [specific deadline within 2 weeks]. Thanks so much.*

Go on – do it. You will *not* regret it.


## DISCOVERING AND LIVING MY VALUES

*'Don't ask what the world needs. Ask what makes you come alive, and go do it. Because what the world needs is people who have come alive.'* Howard Thurman

Values are quite simply (and quite profoundly) what's most important to us. We may feel irritability, disconnection or even anguish if our values are ignored or overridden. And when we get to live and work in a place of alignment with our values we feel alive and engaged; we flourish.

*'Knowing my values changes everything. I can now feel liberated in making decisions because I know what's guiding them. I have a clearer sense of what I am saying yes to and when to say no.'*
Elizabeth, midwife

For example, I have a strong value of harmony. It comes partly from my childhood as middle sister of three girls: I'm the one who seeks to bridge the gap. And therefore when I'm in disharmony or conflict with someone I feel out of sorts and my energy is drained. I will seek to restore harmony where I can, as harmony creates a feeling of flow or aliveness in me. There is an overlap too with my values of connection and intimacy. I want to feel deeply connected to the people with whom I spend my time, and mostly I want to have real conversations (with raucous laughter and real feeling) about things that matter. Knowing my values means it makes *sense* to me that I am more suited to being in a team than rotating as a midwife with constantly changing patterns of people. I also have strong values of possibility and creativity. When they are trampled by a system or a person saying 'it's just the way it is' or 'who do you think you are thinking that you can...?' I feel a sensation of tightness in my body; a part of me is being stifled.

Our values are so fundamental to who we are that when they are being dishonoured by ourselves or others it can almost feel as if our atmosphere changes: there is less oxygen available to breathe.

If we were a tree, our values would be our roots, the things that keep us anchored when the storm comes, and largely hidden, dig deep into the soil to find the nutrients needed for life. The branches, leaves, flowers or fruit are the expression of our values in the world and for the world.

For all of us, journeying through tough midwifery training is an expression of our values. Compassion, determination and justice come to mind immediately as personal values which have sparked many a midwifery fire, and have the capacity to keep us in the game. Yet we know we're at sea (or at least off the path!) when, hard pressed, we feel disengaged from the woman or family in our care, or become passive, taking a stance of, 'well there's not much I can do'. We might find we are compromising our value of integrity ('I can't align what I believe is right, with what I say and do on a busy postnatal ward'), dignity ('I didn't stand up to that colleague who acted without appropriate consent') or tolerance ('I left that stereotyping of the woman unquestioned at handover').

It's energy-draining, life-draining to be working in a way that

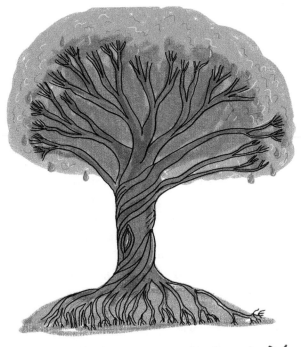

# YOU'RE REALLY
## RATHER BEAUTIFUL

dishonours our values. And energy-giving, life-affirming to honour our values in our life and work. It's easier to feel seen and heard too, because when what we believe and what we do aligns and 'makes sense', people notice.

You may see or hear yourself already in these examples. The list below is purely for reference as you work through the six values-mining exercises below. Values can't easily be picked from a list without context. Instead, the exercises highlight the living nature of these words in you. When you land on one that's really true for you there is a resonance – a feeling of vibration, depth and 'right-ness', usually felt in the body as well as the mind.

## LIST OF VALUES

(adapted from Brené Brown, *Dare To Lead* 2019)[2]

| | | | |
|---|---|---|---|
| Accountability | Ethics | Justice | Self-respect |
| Achievement | Excellence | Kindness | Serenity |
| Adaptability | Fairness | Knowledge | Service |
| Adventure | Faith | Leadership | Simplicity |
| Altruism | Family | Learning | Spirituality |
| Ambition | Financial stability | Legacy | Sportsmanship |
| Authenticity | Forgiveness | Leisure | Stewardship |
| Balance | Freedom | Love | Success |
| Beauty | Friendship | Loyalty | Teamwork |
| Being the best | Fun | Making a difference | Thrift |
| Belonging | Future generations | Nature | Time |
| Career | Generosity | Openness | Tradition |
| Caring | Giving back | Optimism | Travel |
| Collaboration | Grace | Order | Trust |
| Commitment | Gratitude | Patience | Truth |
| Community | Growth | Patriotism | Understanding |
| Compassion | Harmony | Peace | Uniqueness |
| Competence | Health | Perseverance | Usefulness |
| Confidence | Home | Personal fulfillment | Vision |
| Connection | Honesty | Power | Vulnerability |
| Contentment | Hope | Pride | Wealth |
| Contribution | Humility | Recognition | Well-being |
| Cooperation | Humour | Reliability | Wholeheartedness |
| Courage | Inclusion | Resourcefulness | Wisdom |
| Creativity | Independence | Respect | |
| Curiosity | Initiative | Responsibility | Write your own: |
| Dignity | Integrity | Risk -taking | ................... |
| Diversity | Intimacy | Safety | ................... |
| Environment | Intuition | Security | ................... |
| Efficiency | Job security | Self-discipline | ................... |
| Equality | Joy | Self-expression | ................... |

## VALUES MINING SWEET-SIX

### I. A peak moment in time to discover my values: a solo or partner exercise

This is a chance to have a close and delightful look at a peak moment when life was especially rewarding or poignant. It's important that it is a 'moment' or an 'event' otherwise there may be too much information to sift through to find the core values. You can do this on your own, reading the script, listening to the script at <u>flourishformidwives.com</u> and then answering the questions. Or even better, involve a partner.

*Take a few moments to settle into your body... begin to notice the rhythm of your breath... the rise and the fall of your chest. Enjoy the sensation of allowing your breath to flow... Feel the softness in your face and your shoulders with each out breath... Let the breath and that softness go all the way to your belly... Notice the sound of your breath, in and out, and then bring your awareness to any sounds in the room or in your environment. Just notice them, and then come back to your softening breath.*

*Now cast your mind to a time in your life when you felt fully alive, so alive that you were almost vibrating with the energy of just being you. Join in the scene as if it's happening right now: what or who you can see? Notice the colours, the shapes, the weather, the light. What can you hear? Reach out and touch something. What textures or temperatures do you notice? What can you smell in this place? Breathe that in... let it all come so alive for you right now that you can almost taste it.*

Slowly come back into the present, and in the quiet jot down as much detail from the experience as you want. Then gently ask yourself the following questions (or ask a partner to):

- What was happening?
- Who was there?
- What else did you notice?
- What was your part/your impact?
- What were the values that were being honoured in that moment?
- What does 'X' (Name the value) mean to you?

Additional questions/prompts for a partner to ask you:

- Is there a value of X (name the value you are guessing) or Y in that experience?
- It sounds like you were honouring a value around X. Does that sound right? (There will be a more tangible verbal or non-verbal reaction when the words ring true.)
- What does 'X' (name the value) mean to you?

Write down the values that come out as strong/clear/resonant for you.

## 2. Peak midwifery moment

One of the absolute stand-out moments of my midwifery training, one which still makes me glow, was a moment on antenatal ward. A pregnant woman with a toddler at home had shown signs of pre-term labour so had become a 'resident' for a couple of weeks for twice daily CTGs and reviews. On her toddler's second birthday we not only arranged for her toddler and husband to join her for a mini party, but also managed to talk her out of her room for long enough to decorate it, source and wrap beautiful new gifts from the cupboard on the paediatric ward and find a cake. Her joy on seeing all of this was deeply rewarding. Party over, she went on to birth her new baby safely at the end of that same day. In that moment, I was able to honour my values of resourcefulness, initiative, collaboration and 'home'. Home sounds like a strange thing to call a value, but I have long been motivated by the desire to bring a sense of 'home' to the people I care for wherever they are, so I guess it's a value for me.

Use the script above in exercise 1 and try this out with your joy-filled midwifery moments, even if they feel far away right now.

## 3. Suppressed values

Another way to name your values is to isolate a moment when you felt frustrated, distressed or angry. Often this will signal a value that is being suppressed. Because we are often choosing to honour our values in life without even being aware of it, it's sometimes easier to recognise them when something gets in the way.

Try it out:

- Briefly name the situation when you were distressed.
- Take a piece of paper folded into four quadrants.
- Write down the feelings that accompanied the situation.
  One feeling/metaphor for a feeling per quadrant.
- Then turn over the paper and in the corresponding quadrants on
  the other side name what the opposite sensation/desire might be.
  Try it out: you might find a value or two there.

For example, Ayesha writes 'silenced', 'no choices' in two quadrants.
She then flips over her paper and on the corresponding quadrants
writes 'freedom to speak'. There are actually two values here: both
freedom/independence and voice/speaking out.

After more thinking time and prompting from her partner, she
writes in the other two quadrants 'humiliated', 'unvalued'. On the
other side, she writes 'respect'. She's discovering that respect is a huge
value for her personally, and for the culture that she has grown up in.
Disrespect feels almost like physical pain for her. She now has some
knowledge, helping her to discern *why* she is finding certain situations
more challenging than others, and *what* she might need to do or assert
to feel more in alignment with herself next time.

### 4. Must-haves

Must-haves in life are another way to work out your values.

Try it out.

Beyond the fundamentals of nourishment, security and
community, what else must you have for a sense of fulfilment and
aliveness? Is adventure or exploration a must-have for you? What
about a strong thread of creativity in your life or work? What about
your relationships with others? Must you have togetherness and
collaboration? Your chosen environment might be a must-have: must
you have access to nature/mountains/sea/trees? What are the values
you absolutely must honour —or part of you dies?

### 5. Obsessive expression

It is possible for us to begin to insist on a value so much that it mutates into more of a demand. Maybe you've experienced this in others – perhaps when your family member's value of order, or your colleague's value of excellence mutates into a demand for perfection. Perhaps you see it in yourself: when a value of responsibility becomes control, friends and family are quick to point it out! A value of growth or innovation might turn into a hyper-focus on work matters, a value of efficiency might spill into neglecting the human dynamics. There are important values here that are coming out in an extreme or obsessive form. Look for the value, and don't focus on the mutation, extreme or obsessive expression.

Try asking yourself these questions. I have answered for myself to give you some examples

- What do you say about yourself? *I won't settle until...* value = justice or persistence
- What do people tease you about? *That I'm 'keen' (read obsessive):* value = activism or change
- What drives friends or family nuts about you? *That I'm controlling:* value = responsibility

### 6. Values playground

Now that you have more of a values vocabulary, try answering the questions below (expanded from a set in *Life Reimagined* by Richard Leider and Alan Webber, 2013)[3] and play with how this amplifies the information you already have about your values.

Treat this lightly. Move fairly quickly through each one. Go from your gut. Write down the answers. One-word answers are fine.

- What motivates me to get up in the morning?
- What keeps me up at night? What issues tug at me?
- What am I doing when I'm at my best?
- Why am I bothered by what bothers me?
- Why do I do the work I do?
- Why do I live where I live?
- Why do I buy what I buy?
- Why do I long for what I long for?

- Why do I read and watch what I do?
- Why do I admire whom I admire?
- When am I most content?
- Why do I choose the relationships that I choose?

Now gather together your top five values from *all* six exercises and write them down. *Don't skip this bit.*

Then reflect on the questions below for each value. Each one will deepen your connection to your values:

- When or how was I taught the importance of this value? (Something you 'picked up', or from direct lessons)
- What feelings come up for me when I think about this value?
- Is this value really mine? (This is looking out for the dangerous and not-you 'I *should* think this, feel this, want this…') Test it out with these juicy questions from Jo Bradshaw.
  - If you weren't allowed to do this/express this anymore, what would you miss most?
  - And what internal promise would you be breaking?
  - Would you fight for this (think visceral)?[4]
- Write your list of five values in a left-hand column. For each value, name an example of a time when it was being fully honoured (lived) or dishonoured (trampled – by you or others)

| Value | Dishonoured | Fully honoured |
| --- | --- | --- |
| | | |
| | | |
| | | |
| | | |

In what specific ways (activities/pursuits) can I live my five most important values now?

## 551 ME AS AN INSTRUMENT IN AN ORCHESTRA – MY VOICE AND WHAT I BRING

You don't have to have experience of playing in an orchestra to imagine the swell of the music around you. Try this out:

*Get settled, focus for 30 seconds just on your breath... and then picture yourself in among an orchestra as if the orchestra were a group of colleagues/your wider team/your wider family. Notice where you are sitting. Notice which instrument you are playing. What is it about that instrument, particularly the sound/tone or character of that instrument, that reflects who you are? What can you say about how your voice plays a role in relation to others in the orchestra? Notice the impact of your instrument on the overall sound, when it chooses to come 'in' and when it stays silent.*

*If you could move seats right now and choose another instrument (assuming that you are just as technically gifted there too!), what would you choose? What is it about this instrument, its sound, tone or character, that reflects who you are but don't show so often?*

*How do your chosen instrument(s) reflect your values?*

*Notice whether imagining the orchestra as a work team or wider family makes a difference to the instrument you choose, how/when you use it in relation to others, and the impact it has on the overall sound.*

The instrument that reflects most closely my vibe and the impact of my voice is a bass clarinet. It's quite deep and soulful, not brassy but somewhat distinctive in its size at over a metre long. It looks a little like a saxophone but is not trying to be one. It plays the bass line, which can make others in the orchestra feel secure and held. It often plays its part on its own, unlike the soprano clarinets, so is more likely to be heard when others are quiet or reflective. It also has the capacity to 'still' others, so it can bring a team into that place of quiet.

As a coach and as a midwife, I am aware that my bass clarinet voice is a natural one for me. I am aware of the gifts it brings, not least that it already has a wide range of sound. And depending on the day and who I am working with, I work to expand my 'range' to the arresting directness of trumpet or the gentle lift of flute or the playfulness of first violin.

What are you learning about your voice, its dynamics and its relationship with others from this exercise? Journal about it or discuss with your partner.

## RECALLING THE DREAM

So you came into midwifery with a picture of how life would be and how you would be able to make your contribution to the world. How easy does it feel to recall that picture?

Purpose is good for us.[5] It gives our lives a sense of coherence, and helps us to self-regulate feelings, set goals and make good health choices. The Japanese concept of *ikigai*, often translated as 'a reason for being' has, lived out, been shown to increase life expectancy.[6] While this Venn diagram is a distortion of the real meaning of *ikigai* – the small, significant, often personal or humble pursuit of doing something you enjoy[7] – it does help us define purpose in this moment.

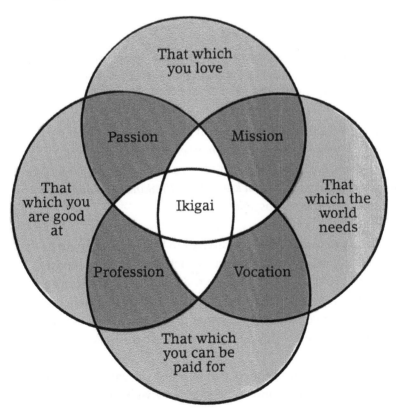

Marc Winn's 2014 Venn diagram overlaid onto the concept of ikigai[8]

Note down below what you remember of your original midwifery dream. If it helps, think about the longing to serve (that which the world needs) and the passion that you brought (that which you love). Maybe pull out old promises you made to yourself, or a university application. Note and celebrate if there are elements of it that you are currently living.

Don't worry if you get stuck. The exercises below are designed to lead us back to our sense of purpose step by step.

.......................................................................................................

.......................................................................................................

.......................................................................................................

.......................................................................................................

.......................................................................................................

.......................................................................................................

This is what I wrote in a blog on International Day of the Midwife 2017, as I entered the world of midwifery. I can go back to it and use it to recapture that spirit of focus.

> 'This is the high dream: that I might use all of who I am made to be – the woman, the voice, the mother, the coach – to bring refreshment and possibility to midwives who are losing hope. I am not one to hold back, as you know, from thinking deep and wide, believing anything is possible.'

We are going to use a series of exercises to help recall and revive your sense of purpose in the world – which you can then choose to use in midwifery – or elsewhere if that's a better place for you. The visualisations below are best listened to, so access them on flourishformidwives.com, get a partner to read them one by one, or record them yourself with lots of pauses where the dots are, and then listen back.

You can do all of this sequence in one session, with a notebook or paper in front of you for quiet note-taking between each one.

## REDISCOVERING MY SENSE OF PURPOSE

*Come into your body by focusing on your feet on the floor, your bottom or back well supported. When you are ready, start to notice the rhythm of your breath... the cool of the in-breath... and the warmth as the breath comes out... notice the rise and the fall of your chest, as you feel your shoulders and your face softening with every out breath... Focus for a few breaths on the out-breath and notice how any parts of your body which are tight – your hands, your jaw... your thighs... can be eased or softened by focusing on them and letting the out-breath soften the muscles... Then focus on the in-breath. Notice the oxygen that you take in with that conscious in-breath. Watch it in your mind's eye travel around your body, fuelling every cell, bringing a sense of aliveness to your limbs, your fingers and toes... You are about to be transported to some curious places. Stay gently in your body and just let your mind follow...*

### Visualisation 1 – 90th birthday party

*It's your 90th birthday and you're wonderfully vital in your old age. There's a party in the garden of your home. Lots of people have come from your whole life (it's a magical party and everyone's there including people who may have already died) – family, friends, people you've enjoyed working with... You're sitting enjoying all these people you are fond of as they enjoy the party... just watch them interact... notice the colours... the sounds... the feeling of the atmosphere... Listen now as they talk to each other. What are they saying about what you've meant to them?... One of them comes over, gives you a hug and thanks you for transforming their life... Really listen to them: what was it about what you did and who you are that has had such an impact on them?...*

### Visualisation 2 – billboard and message

*Picture a busy road in a city near you, the kind of large road so busy that cars will regularly have to slow down enough to take in what's around them. You have just been given free maxi billboard space on that road. Thousands of people pass by it every day. You have the opportunity to impact these people in any way you choose. What would you put on that billboard?... Which colours would you use?... See it now... What are the images?... What's your message for the world?... Now picture the people in the cars slowing down and taking it in as they pass... What's the impact on them?... What's being touched or shaped in them right now because of your message?*

### Visualisation 3 – miracle morning

*Something beautiful happened overnight: you've been given an extraordinary gift. As you wake today you feel changed, with power and energy moving through your body... feel that aliveness now as you breathe... You choose to go out, walk among others and share some of this gift... imagine yourself now in a thronging crowd... you notice the people you feel drawn to reaching out and touching... look at their faces... those who you touch are transformed completely and wonderfully... who do you choose to touch?... what is the impact of your touch?... What is the gift?*

### Visualisation 4 – future self

*You're at a large gathering hearing the buzz of conversation and the clink of glasses. Your future self is up on a stage. Take a really good look at this person – what are they wearing, how do they hold themselves, stand or walk?... What atmosphere do they bring into the room? As they begin to speak to the group, you notice their voice. What's appealing about that voice?... What does it create?... You are aware of a shift that is happening to you and everyone around you. Your future self is having a deep impact on you and on others. You are all being profoundly shaped or changed... What is the impact your future self is having on you and the others?... How are you and others transformed?... Who is your future self being to have such an impact?... Notice now the feeling of walking out into the world changed forever. What's that like? What do you want to say, if anything, now to your future self?*

### Visualisation 5 – uninhabited island

*You are getting into a vessel. As you launch, you realise that you are on your way to an uninhabited island, with the scope to create an environment and a community from scratch. You have the power to create this island to be whatever you want it to be. When you land, what is it that you're going to make happen?... What's the impact you want to have?... The vessel is landing on the island. The door opens. You reach down and touch the soil of the island and say, 'It's going to be this way.' What is 'this way'?*

## FINDING MY 'BIG WHY' – RADIATING FROM THE INSIDE OUT

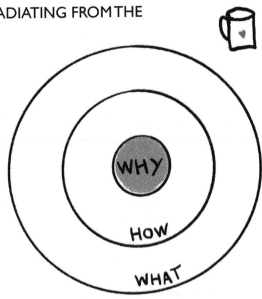

Our 'Big Why' is the heart of why we do what we do, or live as we live. Capturing it can reignite a sense of purpose and agency in our lives. Simon Sinek originally introduced this concept in his book *Start With Why*[9] as a way of describing how effective leaders influence the success of a project, product or organisation: starting *not* with the conventional 'What We Do', or 'How We Do It', but the cause or belief from which everything else flows. We talked in Part I about compassion fatigue. The flip side is compassion satisfaction: the sense of being connected to the care moment and aligned (in terms of values and principles) with who you are choosing to be and what you are choosing to do. Knowing our Big Why can help with this sense of alignment and satisfaction. It can also be a huge motivator for ourselves in the day to day, and for others as we initiate change.

You can watch the talk at www.ted.com/talks/simon_sinek_how_great_leaders_inspire_action then discover your Big Why by exploring the following questions:

- What are your deepest passions?
- What issues in the world do you feel passionately about?
- What about in the midwifery world?
- How does that link to your original dream?
- What rankles you or inspires you?
- What would you be prepared to stand for or against?

Keep it short; try to focus on the thing that stirs you most and keeps you stirred.

Complete this sentence:

*'I want to live in a world where...*

*because it's not okay that...'*

I asked a few midwives, student midwives and maternity support workers to define their Big Why as examples for you:

*'I want to live in a world where women from all different backgrounds have equal access to information, education and fair treatment to empower themselves in healthcare settings. Because it's not ok that Black and Asian women have such bad outcomes due to a lack of caregiver knowledge and good treatment. Every woman deserves excellent care and compassion!'* Dionne, newly-qualified midwife

*'I want to live in a world where early interventions are well funded and readily available for women and their families. Because it's not okay that we don't all have access to the same start in life.'* Effie, midwife

*'I want to live in a world where choice, honesty, and individuality are understood better as no one is the same person or will necessarily have the same outcome. My passion is to give individualised care and support based on choice and offer my unbiased advice and continuity to make a difference in their journey.*

*Because it's not okay that the whole experience for everyone changes course when we don't have enough time to give continued individualised care.'* Karen, MSW

I then asked these people to complete the sentence *'so I'm going to...'* They all said 'I don't know yet...' And that's okay. What they do know, and what I know of them, is that they will continue to take small, significant steps towards equity in access to care, choosing roles where they can wave a banner for the equity, justice and individualised care in maternity that is their heart-cry. Even without knowing the 'what now...?', they are still guided in the day to day, in their smaller and bigger choices, by their Big Why.

Back to you: now that you know your heart-cry or battle-cry... if you could express it to the world on a T-shirt or a banner (probably

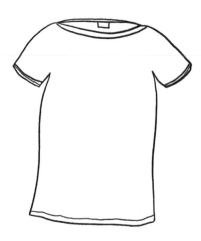

ending with an exclamation mark!), what would it say? Write it down. Remember this doesn't mean you *would* put it on a T-shirt, or that knowing your Big Why necessarily means an outward or vocal kind of activism. It might be a quiet determination for the area you want to steward – the thing that will bring you deep satisfaction. MSW Karen's heart-cry is 'ENCOURAGE!' You can see it all over the way she lives, and the way she longs to practice.

## CREATING MY VISION BOARD/IMAGE

Even those of you not usually tempted by so-called creative pursuits might enjoy the outcome of this exercise. The purpose is to use images, colours and words if you choose, to form a picture or collage of your purpose to serve as a very visual reminder of who you are and what shapes and inspires you. A vintage iteration might involve paper, glue and cut out magazine images or printed photos; less vintage would be making a Pinterest board or creating an Instagram account dedicated to images that feel representative of you. Before you pin or post anything, ask yourself the following two questions:

- What do I like about this image?
- Which significant word or value (for me) does it match up with?

Either way each image – and the overall result – is capturing something of the flavour of you and your distinctive contribution to the world. It is a way of representing all that you've discovered in the exercises above. Many coaching clients over the years have not only enjoyed the process, but been inspired and encouraged by the images for years to come. Have fun!

Here are some examples from my wonderful illustrator Jo: www. pinterest.co.uk/minestronesoul/minestrone-soul-mood-board

And one I created capturing the experience of a coaching journey: www.pinterest.co.uk/wildrubiescoach/ come-on-board-the-dhow-journey

## ONE HUNDRED DREAMS

This is a chance to reactivate your dreaming 'muscles'. Capture as many dreams as you can, in no particular order. Tempting as it may be, don't censor yourself. Perhaps put on some well-loved music and begin to write. Think in terms of what you want to do, what/who you want to be, what you want to have. The dreams could be physical, spiritual, creative, centred on family, emotional, about relationships, professional, financial. Many will be fun. Some will feel adventurous and daring. Others will reflect a simple longing in you... When you slow down or get stuck, ask yourself, 'What else would I love?...' Cast your mind back to previous dreams you have held, and forgotten or discarded. They may or may not feel 'alive' for you anymore, but they may spark some more in your mind. Allow yourself to ponder, to doodle and meander. Remember you will experience a dream drought, probably somewhere around 25, 35, 45, or 55 dreams. It's a really good dream muscle reactivation exercise to keep going. Get up, move around, make a cup of tea, change the mood of the track on the music app, have a shower, go for a run, and let those dreams keep surfacing. Enjoy the freedom it gives you to be audacious. If you remain stuck after all of the above, try these questions as playful prompts:

- What books/ films/songs did you love when you were little?
- What kind of worlds did you build for yourself back then?
- Name something that moves you to tears/joy. Use that to reconnect with lost or censored parts of yourself.

## THE LONG GAME: LETTER FROM FUTURE SELF TO CURRENT SELF

Mentally position yourself in 20 years' time. Write down the date at the top of a piece of paper. Start a letter to you now from you in 20 years' time, with all the wisdom, hindsight and tenderness that you bring for your current self. Start simply and use these prompts if it helps.

*Dear xxxx,*
*I've been wanting to encourage you about what's ahead*

*I've been...*

*What I most want to tell you is...*

*You'll be so happy to hear that...*

*And also...*

*You might be surprised to hear that...*

*What I know now that I didn't know when I was your age is...*

*Love xxxx*

## FINDING MY TRIBE – ALLIES FOR THE JOURNEY

So who's in my tribe and what does that even mean? Your tribe are the mates and soulmates who get you, get on the path with you and are committed to the flourishing of you and your ideas. It could be that some of them are already working through this book with you. Maybe you have a band of midwives from university days who have travelled the winding road together and share values or dreams. Or perhaps you are now able to actively seek out your tribe based on the discoveries from the exercises in this section of the book. You now know what inspires and motivates you. Others will want the same.

Some strategies for finding your tribe:

- Spot people at work who share a similar frustration or sadness or vision about 'the way things are' and start conversations.
- Use Twitter to connect with people who are choosing a similar path (these algorithms can have their benefits!) Not only that, put out a message on Twitter or any social media platform asking all your mates to connect you with others in their lives who share your passions.
- Actively seek a role that aligns with what and who you want more of in your life – whether it's a continuity team with a focus on vulnerable women, or a role with colleagues or a leader who can be a mentor and see you for who you are.
- Remember that your people are not necessarily your peers. Ask for mentors where you find them. Making requests like this is an excellent example of vulnerability showing up as courage and is almost always welcome.

See p.217 for ways to get your tribe involved in your 'small change, big impact' project.

## SABOTAGE! SEEING, HEARING AND RESPONDING TO MY 'SABOTEUR' VOICES

Saboteurs are the voices in our heads seeking to keep us 'safe'. In fact they started life with us as children as 'guardians' helping us fend off physical and emotional threats, whether real or imagined. As adults, you could argue we no longer have need for them. But as Shirzad Chamine of Positive Intelligence says, 'they have become invisible inhabitants of our mind',[10] automating default patterns for responding to known and unknown situations. They do this by repeating old stories or mantras, usually to maintain our 'safety', keep us small or even invisible. Many of their sentences might start with the phrase, 'For your own good, may I suggest that you...?'

'Why on earth would you want to risk putting yourself out there?' one of your saboteurs might ask. One of the ones I hear most often comes out waving a flag with this tone '(loud cough)... Just saying, if you don't control this situation, it might start to control you'. Ouch. Can you hear how (relatively) kindly and polite it is? But also how it is setting off a fear-based alarm system in me which screams that the alternative to control is chaos or being controlled. So these voices or characters can end up causing anxiety, self-doubt and frustration in us, and sabotage (hence the name) our relationships and the way we show up in the world.

NB: Saboteur voices will likely shout/whisper more insistently when we are stepping out/moving towards our purpose.

It's really helpful to know where yours pop up, what they might say and how they are seeking to 'save' you from your best self. In coaching when a saboteur appears, as they frequently do, we redirect in one of two ways, either:

- shine an ultra-bright light on them, find out exactly who they are and what they look like, zoom in on their tone of voice and what they are saying. This tends to expose them as saboteurs as opposed to voices of reason. The newly gained clarity often reveals how alarmist and fairly ridiculous they are. The person can then respond to the saboteur with the truth (rather than the lie) about what's really called for in this moment.
- bypass the saboteur and go straight to a person's values and purpose. In this moment the person knows there is nothing to fear and everything to play for. The saboteur knows they have been trumped and instantly quietens.

You can do a free assessment of your saboteur voices at www.positiveintelligence.com/saboteurs

Shirzad Chamine[11] names 10 saboteur voices: the judge, the hypervigilant, the hyperachiever, the avoider, the controller, the restless, the stickler (perfectionist), the victim, the pleaser, the hyperrational. In reality there could be any number of variations, but this assessment is an excellent way in. Write down the following:

*My main saboteur's name is...*

*My saboteur is fond of saying or often says...*

*Now I know this saboteur I want to reply with this...*

It's also good to note of course that saboteurs can show up in a family or organisational culture as well as in an individual. Try completing this sentence:

*Inside my organisation/community/family, these saboteur comments sometimes show up...*

Discuss this with a trusted partner or group. Share how your saboteur shows up at work and how you are now choosing to respond to it. Use a journal or phone note to record moments when the saboteur appears and, without unleashing 'the judge' saboteur, what you choose to do.

NB. Saboteurs never completely go away. You just learn to notice and then manage them more effectively. Their voices can definitely quieten or just start to sound irrelevant!

## PASSION AND PURPOSE SUMMARY: THE STORY OF ME WALK

Try completing the prompts below. Or try it another way. Do a Story of Me walk first and then complete the prompts.

Meet with your trusted partner for a walk in a quiet place, and agree that you will spend 20 minutes just talking about you and what you've been discovering, and being listened to. Set an alarm so you don't have to check the clock. You keep talking, and your partner keeps listening, with no comment, intervention, attempt to encourage or rescue. When you feel like the words have dried up, let the silence be there. There is more, it just needs the space of the silence to emerge. Then reflect, as the speaker, on what it was like to be listened to in that way. What emerged that you didn't expect? What have you discovered even in the process of talking about yourself? And for the listener, what was it like for you to listen like that? What impulses did you need to resist as you continued to listen? What are you learning about yourself? Take some time before you swap over into listening mode to record what you noticed:

*What have I discovered about*

- *myself*
- *my dreams*
- *my values*
- *my purpose in the world and in midwifery*
- *my saboteurs*
- *my tribe and what they care about?*

*What am I noticing about the stories I keep telling myself?*

*Who would I be without that storyline?*

# CHAPTER 14

# IN THE WHOLE OF LIFE

*'I went from a person who was frequently described as strong and independent to a person whose entire life was taken over by stress, anxiety and depression. It took many, many months of treatment and inner reflection to rebuild my identity and sense of self-worth. I am a different person now to who I was when I became a midwife. I've had to reckon with some painful truths about my profession, my boundaries and myself to get to the place I am now, as a much stronger, wiser and more self-assured woman who knows what she is capable and worthy of, and what she won't tolerate or do.'* Amity Reed, midwife[1]

These 'in the whole of life' exercises or practices are designed to help you begin to curate a stronger self-awareness and sense of choice as to how to respond to the tsunamis of life and the daily body blows of midwifery. We know from research that true resilience starts with self-awareness. Audre Lorde spoke of what has been stolen from Black women, the love for each other, using these words: 'We have to study how to be tender with each other until it becomes habit'. She adds 'We can practice being gentle with each other by being gentle with that piece of ourselves that is hardest to hold.'[2]

This is not about some kind of wishy-washy notion of tenderness and self-care. Bubble baths as a go-to have their place, don't get me wrong: they can wash away some of the emotional grime of the day and go some way towards soothing intolerable feelings. But there is still a question of what we do with those feelings when we get out of the bath; how we learn to listen or choose differently, and have courageous conversations with ourselves and others as we advocate for something better. This is radical self-care (in its original meaning of rooted, rooting, fundamentally grounding). This goes 'beyond kale and pedicures' in the words of Françoise Mathieu of the TEND institute,[3] wholesome and feel-good as they are. This recognises that while soothing 'strategies' may act like a sea wall, holding back the impact of the waves, a deeper approach is to cultivate our soothing system and way of being that includes our vulnerability.

Yes this is an invitation, in life and in our work to learn to be with our

- Not knowing
- Imperfections
- Vulnerabilities (from the Latin word 'to wound')

and model them in our leadership, in work and in our families.

As Brené Brown, social worker and researcher into shame and vulnerability, says in *The Gifts of Imperfection*:

*'Owning our own story can be hard, but not nearly as difficult as spending our lives running from it. Embracing our vulnerabilities is risky, but not nearly as dangerous as giving up on love and belonging and joy - the experiences that make us most vulnerable. Only when we are brave enough to explore the darkness will we discover the infinite power of light.'*[4]

Vulnerability is not weakness. In fact it's the opposite. Vulnerability is our strongest and most authentic state; a state of being aware of ourselves and open, both to wounding and also to joy.

And vulnerability opens the window for the fresh air of self-compassion which asks the question 'What do I need right now – to alleviate my suffering so that I can go on bringing myself to serve the world and its needs?'. The research of Kristin Neff shows clearly that when we are better equipped to be compassionate towards ourselves, we are more able to show compassion to others. She draws the distinction between tender self-compassion (being with ourselves, including with our pain, in an accepting way, including soothing and reassuring ourselves) and fierce self-compassion, which is more 'active' and might involve clearly drawing boundaries, standing tall or fighting an injustice.[5] Both are needed.

So take time over these exercises with yourself, your chosen partner or your mini group. Start exploring what shifts physically and emotionally for you when you bring these practices into life for the next few days and weeks.

## CHECK IN TO START: THE THREE CIRCLES

Paul Gilbert's Compassion Focused Therapy three circles model[6] helps us frame what we are doing here. Look at the circles model. The Drive System, our get up and go system, can be highly activated in many of us – which while exciting and rewarding, can be exhausting if it is not in balance with the Soothe System, and can even tip over into activating the Threat System. You can see how easily how an overactive drive and threat system (both in principle working for good – to spur us on, and to alert us to hazards including the threat of rejection or isolation) can lead to burnout, especially in the absence of ways of being that bring us back to a place of regulation and wellbeing. The BBC screen adaptation of Adam Kay's *This is Going to*

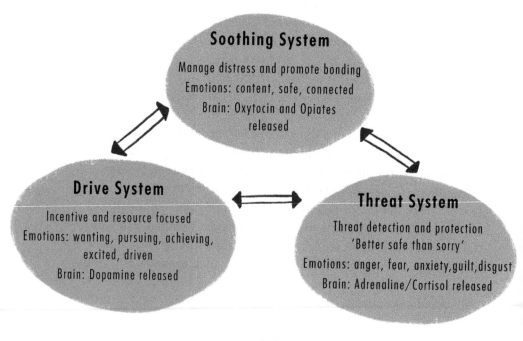

*Hurt*[7] showed us a set of high drive medics operating in a high threat environment with no soothing mechanisms, leading to deep suffering. The systems work best when they are in balance.[8]

Draw your own version of the circles, in different sizes, according to your current balance between the three. Do it without judgement, just noticing what feels larger or smaller for you right now.

Both our drive and soothe systems can help regulate the threat system. It's one of the reasons why taking action (drive system) can feel good in the midst of fear or anxiety. If your threat system is like a bike catapulting down a hill, imagine your soothe system in particular as like a set of brakes. How can you deploy it to reduce the sense of threat in the moment and move more easily into a helpful state of problem-solving or creativity?

Here are some quick ideas which correspond with the principles in the exercises below of move the body and breath, move the mind.

- Use a grounding technique – really *feeling* your feet inside your shoes, noticing the feeling of fabric on skin; or try placing your hands on something of a different temperature, like the counter in a labour room, or the outside of a water bottle, and feeling them for 30 seconds.
- Breathe rhythmically for two minutes – in for a count of four and out for a count of four.
- Thank the threat system for its help – a similar approach as speaking directly to our saboteurs – see p.160. Simply saying 'Thank you for your help, I don't need you right now' can be enough to shift the focus away from the activated limbic system and put on the brakes.

## MOVE THE BODY: MINISTERING TO THE BODY AS A DISCIPLINE – WHAT'S IN MY WEEK?

What's in my week that gets me into my body or directly soothes, strengthens or supports my body? One of the challenges of shift work, particularly rotating shift work, is unpredictable schedules, taking their toll on rhythms in our lives. In Part I we highlighted the crashing impact of circadian rhythm disruption, but we are also talking about the disruption to the kinds of daily rhythms which enable us to use and soothe our bodies. It is the greatest irony, many would say, that to practise midwifery effectively we need to be 'occupying' our own bodies, to enable a woman to step closer to being fully in hers.

What happens to our midwifery practice then when we neglect our bodies? I can tell you what happens to mine – I feel less grounded, more exposed, less present in the moment, more vulnerable to veering off course (dishonouring my values). What happens to you?

In your journal, working solo or with your partner, map out your ideal week. Use a different colour if that appeals for each element of your week. Envision what you *really want* – don't hold back – even if your current reality looks or feels different with a rota (or a gang of young children) smashing your ideal world to smithereens. This might include work time, connection time with friends or family, time in nature, time alone, time playing music/reading/pursuing interests. Also include:

- space for exercise/movement
- space for pausing, reflecting and pottering – even if it's just one hour set aside on one free (or childcare available) morning a week.

Remember this is to increase your sense of intentionality. It doesn't matter if your week ends up looking exactly like this at any point, ever. The reality, which I've seen with hundreds of coaching clients over the years, is that defining your week shapes your decisions. Deciding that, even in the midst of a crazy unpredictable rota, you will choose movement or exercise for three hours a week means it is more likely to happen and gives you a sense of clarity as you plan the week or day ahead.

Choose to take whatever action you need to create your space for exercise/movement. Remember some of this could be with children, getting outdoors. Don't be restricted by notions of what it has to look like. Also take action to create space for pausing and pottering.

Commit to accountability with a supportive partner or group. 'I'm going to...' Write it down. Remember: it's all about getting into your body, or doing what directly soothes, strengthens or supports your body, which then serves the whole of you.

Side benefits of this delicious ideal week exercise might be:

- Beginning to see where and how many midwifery hours work best for you. Don't panic: new conversations and possibilities will come out of this.
- Refocusing you on your interests and what most relaxes you.
- Deciding what to say no to (it's not in the map of the week).
- Deciding with more clarity what to say yes to. Oh yeah! (That kind of yes...)

Ask yourself:

- What am I choosing to stop now?
- What do I intend to start now?
- What is the story I've been telling myself? What's the glimmer of a new story?

## MOVE THE BODY: POWER PAUSES CHANGE LIVES

One of the reasons we focused above on the space for pausing and pottering is because it is so hard to do. Most of the time we find ourselves on autopilot, gripped by routines, habitual ways of thinking and patterns of behaviour.

So the next body move is an invitation, whatever we are doing, to just stop and notice, to stop and listen, or to move/walk/act (stopping our habitual ways) and notice/listen. I'm calling it a power pause. This isn't a passive thing – it can be done even in a 'busy' situation, with our children or with a woman in labour, as we choose to awaken our senses to what's there in that moment.

Try this out first on your own or with a partner.

Choose an activity you enjoy that involves the senses (most do!) like cooking, or walking in the park, eating, drinking a glass of wine or the first coffee of the day, knitting, dancing, having sex, enjoying a beautiful view. Take and release a deep breath. Feel your feet and the presence of your whole body. Take another breath. With exquisite attention to the detail, ask yourself, what do I see?... and notice... what do I hear?... and notice... what am I touching with any part of me?...

and notice... what do I smell?... and notice...what am I tasting?... and notice...

Pam England, in her book and methodology *Birthing from Within*,[9] suggests a version of this for birthing women and families, using and sensing with the words 'Seeing, Hearing, Touch, Breath' (always back to the breath). She is reminding us all that with practice, even in situations we find really intense – like the height of a full-on contraction, the eye of a toddler's tantrum, the shifting sands of an emergency – we can be in the present moment. This is not 'time out', a separation from the moment, but a practice of being more present in the moment and less caught up with the shadows of past (if only I'd...) or future (what will happen if...) thinking.

If you like it, keep trying this active sensing in situations you enjoy. Then try to do the same as a power pause at work, when you are feeling overwhelmed. Notice what happens in your body and brain when you mentally say and physically feel 'Seeing, Hearing, Touch, Breath'.

## MOVE THE BODY: POWER POSES CHANGE LIVES

The headline here is: changing our bodies changes our minds. Tiny tweaks in our body posture, even temporarily, affect our physiology, how others perceive us and eventually, how we feel about ourselves.

Potentially intimidating situations like the ward round, a job interview, facing a racist comment, in fact any time when we are tempted to feel small or smaller than others in life, creates a body response: a body posture that perpetuates the emotion affecting our mind in that moment, one of weakness or powerlessness or trying to get it right but not sure we will. There is robust evidence to show that when we adopt a pose which makes us feel more powerful – an expansive posture where we take up more space in the room – not only do we feel more powerful, but there is a positive influence on our presence in the room, as perceived by others, as well as our emotions, mood recovery, positive versus negative memory recall, and our own feelings about ourselves.[10,11]

Seems too good to be true? Try it out now. Watch Amy Cuddy's 20-minute 2012 TED talk Your Body Language May Shape Who You

Are at www.youtube.com/watch?v=Ks-_Mh1QhMc

Then try this: picture a place where you feel smaller than your normal self – maybe it's at your partner's parents' place, or in an environment where you feel unsure, a classroom or a social situation. Imagine yourself there now. Picture the setting more closely, note the colours, the sounds, any other people around. Notice either in your mind's eye or sense in your body itself what position or posture your body moves into in this place, this space? What's it like to be here? Notice what sensations are here in your body in this 'smaller' place?

Now experiment with physically unfolding your body into an expansive pose, with your arms or legs wide or your chest open. Feel the sensations in your body now. What do you notice? Stay there – and notice how the sensations evolve. Then imagine yourself back in that room, that uncomfortable place. Maintain the expansive posture, and notice what it's like for you to be there now. What are the signals in your body that something is different? How are others responding to you coming from a different place? If you notice yourself retreating in your body or your mind to smallness, just observe that, and without judgement come back into an unfolded position. Notice how easily you did that, or how it felt hard. It's all just information.

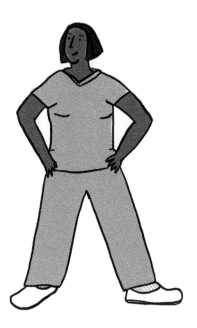

Now try it out in a real life place by giving yourself, as Amy Cuddy suggests, two minutes in a 'power pose' before a challenging situation. Notice what happens.

## MOVE THE BODY: EASY BODY PRACTICE – TREE VISUALISATION

Lots of people love this visualisation. It's also a power pose of a sort, and once we've tried it and felt it, it's a way of connecting quickly with our values and strength.

Try this standing.

*Take a deep breath and shake out your body to ease and loosen your muscles. As you breathe, allow your awareness to drop down into your body. Feel your breath enter and leave your body. Find your own rhythm with your breathing. Settle in and feel the soles of your feet in contact with the floor, ground or your shoes. Imagine your feet growing roots, winding deep down into the soil like a tree with years of wisdom. Feel those roots now, anchoring you and taking up all the nutrients and energy you need... slow and deepen your breath now as you sink down into that sensation of the richness of the soil of your life... As you drink from that soil, feel your heart beating and the sensation of the oxygen flowing through your blood to every cell... sense the aliveness in your body in this moment. Your body is like the trunk of the tree, a channel of intense communication and knowledge. Feel that sensation of standing tall like the tree... Notice what all that upward energy is expanding into. Open up your arms or feel the upward and outward energy of the tree extending into the area around you with branches and lush green leaves. These are the fruit of who you are – what you give and show to the world. Perhaps it is spring and there are flowers there too. Notice what your tree is proudly giving or showing to the world... Notice what it's like to feel alive and refreshed in this moment. And notice the perspective from the height of the tree on your world right now... Know that you have access to this sensation of aliveness and connectedness at any point.*

## MOVE THE BODY: BODY SCAN (Long or short – both work!)

You all know what a body scan is. This is just a reminder of how helpful a gradual, mindful progression of awareness through the body can be, with tension release step-by-step, usually from the feet to the head. You can find body scan-type relaxations in many places including on the Headspace app. If you want a longer version from a trusted source John Kabat-Zinn's Mindfulness Based Stress Reduction Programme's week 1 audio 45-minute body scan is at www.youtube.com/watch?v=UDxJvCZaUAM.

We can't stop the waves in life or in the NHS, but as John Kabat-Zinn said:

> 'You can't stop the waves... but you can learn to surf.' [12]

## MOVE THE BREATH: CHANGE BREATH

We all have moments when negativity or surprise hit us. A change breath is a simple way to stop ourselves reacting to the impact. This exercise and the ones below promote diaphragmatic breathing, stimulating the vagus nerve, improving vagal tone and allowing the parasympathetic nervous system to do its job of soothing. It can be done wherever we are.

> 'Between stimulus and response there is a space. In that space is our power to choose our response. In our response lies our growth and our freedom.' Victor Frankl

Follow these simple steps:

1. Stand upright with your back straight. Put one palm on your belly if you can.
2. Take a slow deep breath in. As you do this, picture clean air entering and filling your whole body. With your in-breath, pull the cleansing air down into your belly and feel your rib cage expand.
3. Take a slow breath out. Picture all toxins or any negativity leaving your body and observe your belly pull in as you fully exhale.
4. Repeat if needed.

## MOVE THE BREATH: BALANCING BREATH

This is a great breath for when we are feeling under pressure. It's quick to do, a little more obvious than the change breath, but easily done. It uses just one hand (thumb and one finger) so could in theory be done with a pen in the other hand. You may laugh at me suggesting we do it in front of the labour ward board, or when our partner or children make us want to scream or shout, but let's model this stuff to each other, to our own families or to the families we are working with. It's incredibly reassuring for them (all) to know that we are looking after ourselves.

1. Close the left nostril with your left thumb.
2. Breathe in deeply and slowly through your right nostril, receiving the breath all through your body.
3. Hold your breath and close the right nostril with your left forefinger.
4. Hold both nostrils closed for a moment.
5. Gently release the thumb from your left nostril and breathe out slowly, keeping your right nostril closed.
6. Take a deep breath through your left nostril, keeping your right nostril closed.
7. Hold both nostrils closed for a moment.
8. Release the right nostril and breathe out slowly.
9. Take a few deep breaths and continue with your notes, your conversation or your day.

## MOVE THE BREATH: SQUARE BREATH OR BOX BREATH

Some people love this breath regulation exercise as it is so visual and so simple. It's also possible to do it easily in the presence of others or in the midst of a stressful situation.

Picture a square. Breathe in up the left-hand side to a count of four, hold across the top of the square for four, breathe out down the right-hand side

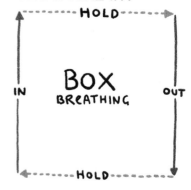

for four and rest for four across the bottom of the square to return to your original position. Repeat until you feel re-centred.

## MOVE THE BREATH: *UJAYI* BREATH

This incredibly powerful breathing exercise stimulates the vagus nerve via the throat and vocal chords, which in turn activates the parasympathetic nervous system and the relaxation response. Using it even for two minutes can be a game-changer when feeling overwhelmed or moving into a panic attack.

If you can, sit with a straight spine and close your eyes. Bring your awareness to your breathing. Breathe in and out in an equal pattern through your nose, with the lips remaining gently closed. As you inhale and exhale, constrict the back of throat, similar to the constriction made when you are speaking in a whisper. In other words, it's an audible, rasping breath, often compared either to the sound of the sea or less poetically to the sound of Darth Vader's voice.

Practice it with your partner or in less stressful situations like preparing to do something difficult, waking up feeling crabby and 'out of sorts' or when stuck in an immovable queue. Notice the profound effect it can have on your body and mind in that moment. You will then have both the incentive and skill to use it when you need it most.

## MOVE THE MIND: RESTORING ME TO WONDER – RECLAIMING THE CONCEPT OF 'FRESH EYES'

*'The most beautiful thing we can experience is the mysterious. It is the source of all true art and all science. He to whom this emotion is a stranger, who can no longer pause to wonder and stand rapt in awe, is as good as dead: his eyes are closed.'* Albert Einstein

The concept of 'fresh eyes', as we all know in midwifery, has been co-opted as part of safety initiatives to 're-look' with a fresh pair of eyes at someone else's assessment, CTG review and so on. I'm going to invite us here to try on a new version of 'fresh eyes'; eyes which look up and look out at the world with a bit more of the white/blue spring-tint lens of the newborn baby, and a bit less of the jaded autumn yellow. This is especially poignant for us as midwives of course as, depending on how we choose to see, we get to witness daily the growth of families and tiny bodies and miraculous birth – and sometimes death, which is also an honour as well as a hardship.

As John O'Donohue asks in his poem 'For the Senses':[13]

*May your soul beautify*
*The desire of your eyes*
*That you might glimpse*
*The infinity that hides*
*In the simple sights*
*That seem worn*
*To your usual eyes*

This takes away nothing of our cries for change: more staff; more care; more pay. What it does is to make available a gift of choosing to see and delight in the wonder of what is in front of us, from the freckle pattern on my youngest daughter's nose to the brilliance of the female body birthing a baby in all its power.

Experiment with your partner, group or journal for one week of making wonder a daily practice. Look for the magic in the ordinary things, or the things that have become commonplace. Pause to be delighted by the sound of your friend's voice in a message. Listen to a piece of inspiring music on your way to work, notice the tiny markers day by day of the changing of the season. Write down one thing per day you have chosen to notice.

Observe what shifts in you when you look differently.

## MOVE THE MIND: GRATITUDE AND ITS POWER

Closely linked to wonder is gratitude. This is how Brené Brown defines gratitude from her research: 'Gratitude is an emotion that reflects our deep appreciation for what we value, what brings meaning to our lives, and what makes us feel connected to ourselves and others'.[14] And while gratitude is an emotion, it is the *practice* of gratitude, much like the *practice* of wonder (doing it, saying it, trying it) that enables us to reap its wide and rich benefits – including elevated immune response, lower blood pressure, improved sleep, better decision-making, decreased aggression and enhanced creativity and optimism.[15]

When we are practising gratitude, speaking out or writing down something we are grateful for, we more deeply appreciate the value of it, take more pleasure from it, and then notice it more. I love Robert Emmon's description of the benefits of practising gratitude: 'Gratitude allows us to participate more in life'.[16] Yes! And while the marketed meme-able version as a cure-all, catch-all 'attitude of gratitude' sells us short, the real thing is juicy and so helpful.

Yes, the real thing fires up our dopamine system, and being grateful towards others makes interacting socially more fun by increasing activation in social dopamine circuits. The real thing boosts serotonin production in the anterior cingulate cortex, by requiring us to look at life's positives. And if there are no positives to be found, in the hardest times of life, it doesn't matter. The very act of searching for *something* to be grateful for appears to affect neuron density in the ventromedial and lateral prefrontal cortex, making it easier to be grateful. Neuroscientist Alex Korb calls it 'The Upward Spiral'.[17]

We have what some researchers have called a 'negativity bias' – designed to keep us safe by remembering hazards or aggression – which affects what sticks. Strong relationships have been shown to need a rough ratio of five positive interactions to one negative; positive memories slip away while hard ones persist, which then shifts our expectations and beliefs towards a more negative bias. And even though hundreds of good things are happening to us and around us every day, we might not see them, notice them or remember them as clearly as we do the negative.

Rick Hanson talks about reorienting this bias by 'tilting toward the good'.[18] This tilt will affect the moment itself by allowing us to really absorb the good thing rather than letting it wash through us and be lost; and the focus on the good, the act of taking it in, will be wiring positive neural structures in our brains. Genius, right? So the handover ritual I mentioned in Part I (see p.114) is partly about tilting towards the good, using appreciative inquiry to tilt us towards what's working, what we've learnt, what we've appreciated in others and in ourselves.

Hanson and team recommend at least a few times each day, when you notice something good, actually letting yourself *feel* good about it, internally, for 20–30 seconds. The longer that we can linger with an awareness of something good, the more neurons fire and wire together, and the stronger we hold traces of that memory.[19] Try it, when you notice something good. See it then feel it. Linger in it if you can. Notice any resistance in you to feeling good and let it pass as you try to really enjoy the experience and sense it filling your body like a warm drink or a glow, becoming an experience which is richer. Later you can journal or get curious about what stories might be behind the fleeting or strong resistance (I don't deserve to feel good, it's selfish to focus on what I have when so much hard stuff is happening in the world, etc etc). For now just enjoy it and know that over time you are weaving a tapestry of positive experiences into the brain's architecture.

## GRATITUDE PRACTICE

So what else might you try?

### *Journaling – on screen or on paper*

Rather than gratitude blitzing (*all* the things/people in your life you are grateful for) aim for a simple practice of recording one thing/person a day you are thankful for. Then write three reasons why. Studies have shown[20,21] that more positive outcomes were experienced by the research group journaling not just what they were grateful for, but the detail of why.

Journaling is an excellent way to capture these daily gratitude notes. Or use a note on your phone, or a gratitude app if you want to enjoy some design or beauty in the process. Message your partner or group with your gratitude what/who and whys every day as another way of recording them, staying on track and enjoying the benefits. If you like things you can touch, write on slips of paper and put them in a gratitude jar along with tickets or notes marking events you were thankful for and want to remember. Empty out the jar at the end of the year and drink in the pleasure. Warning from personal experience: don't keep the jar on a windowsill if you want to be able to read them in 12 months' time. Who would have thought there was so much sun in the UK?!

### Voice messaging or letter writing

Write a letter of gratitude to someone, deliver it to them, and read it to them. Listen to the 'Yours Sincerely' podcast with Jess Phillips MP[22] for inspiration! Or send them a voice message and imagine or listen to their reaction.

### Noticing the one

Make it a practice at work to notice the one: choose one person a day/night to appreciate – be specific if you tell them why.

### Family table round or team check-in

Before dinner, or as you gather as a team, each member of the group says one thing they are grateful for. Watch deeper connection follow (after the derisory teenage snorts have quietened)!

## COMMUTE PRACTICE

This is a what if moment: what if we were to choose to devote the last five minutes of our commute (we know the marker – the stop on the train, or the junction in the car, the point in the road) to naming what we are grateful to be doing rather than what we are dreading? I'm grateful to be seeing colleagues; I'm grateful that there will be someone here tonight who will be my 'one' who I can be extra grateful for; I'm grateful for the opportunity to be with new families as they navigate new territory; I'm grateful for a stocked supply cupboard… This is not about minimising what is unacceptable about the way we work, but choosing to 'tilt towards the good' for the sake of our own and our colleagues' wellbeing.

Start a *wall of gratitude* to remind yourself how what you are doing aligns with who you want to be. By this I am not talking about a wall of any and every card you receive, attractive and feel-good though they are. I'm talking about highlighting or cutting out comments/feedback/images which make you think Yes! This is *why* I do what I do! This is who I want to be as a midwife! I am grateful for this (specifically). This counteracts the 'Thanks so much I couldn't have done it without you, you're an angel' sentiments which although completely heartfelt from parents can make us feel hollow if what we did wasn't necessarily aligned with who we are or who we want to be.

*'And be thankful,'* Colossians 3:15

 ## MOVE THE MIND: THE POWER OF SILENCE IN A NOISY MIDWIFERY WORLD

From the babble of a staff room TV, slam and ping of the microwave, rip of the velcro, crash of the computer on wheels, squeak of ugly shoes on linoleum, jangle of the keys, beep or gallop of the baby's heartbeat, chatter of the nervous parent, insistent alarm of batteries gone, high-pitched squeal of the buzzer, resounding call of the emergency bell, not to mention the sounds of birth or babies…

Through witnessing my youngest daughter's interactions with the world, I am increasingly seeing myself as an HSP (highly sensitive person). Although I manage the stimuli well, I am learning that certain environments drain me quickly, and that the constant noise of a maternity ward is one such place, partly because I'm using energy trying to block out the noise and concentrate. I am also an extrovert. I replenish my energy by being with people and connecting over our ideas and our whole lives, so it's not that I want to go and live in a monastery. It's just that in knowing myself, I know I need to make space in my week to minimise the impact of my draining environments and maximise the opportunity to be in environments that I find uplifting and replenishing. What is a space that uplifts you? If it's a safe place at home (bathroom with door closed), how clear does it need to be of toys/other people's stuff to be your sanctuary? If it's the park or the woods, how far 'in' do you need to go to feel 'away from it'? How can you clearly signal to others – whether at home or out – that you need to be left alone? How could you start asking for what you need?

What's your relationship with silence? What would it mean to make a friend of silence? Write down your ideas. What would it feel like to notice the silences between speech or activities? Try listening for the silence rather than the words. And experiment with leaving empty spaces, either in life or in conversation. What's different when you get to do that?

Write about it or share it with your trusted partner.

## MOVE THE MIND: THE POWER OF WORDS

What language have I been using? What new worlds could I create with new words?

As midwives we seek to understand the impact of our chosen language on the families we care for, and try to choose our words carefully. From the blindingly obvious, insulting and misleading shorthand of 'failure to progress' or 'incompetent cervix', to the slightly more subtle (at least when you explore it in different languages) term 'delivered', suggesting, in English at least, a bizarrely passive role for the person actually birthing the baby. How does it change our whole stance and our communication when we choose to use the word 'decline' positively, with a nod to the freedom to choose enshrined in human rights law? And as midwives, while we likely don't feel as if we have the time to have this conversation, what might change in the consent relationship when we minimise 'let's just pop you on a trace', obscuring the real range of available choices in that moment?[23]

Maybe agree with a trusted partner or group a word or phrase of the month you are all going to try out or 'try on' for size. If you were in a book group, you would come together to discuss your feelings about the book and reactions to it. Try the same for the word or phrase you've been playing with. What's it been like to use it? How has it shaped your conversations or attitude as you consciously substituted this word or phrase in place of another?

Experiment with using these and any others you can think of:

- We *offer* X (screening, foetal monitoring, standardised procedure etc): the following are its limitations… these are possible gains…

it's always your decision.
- We make recommendations, you make *decisions*.
- She *birthed* her baby at 00.23.
- *Optimal cord clamping* (rather than delayed).
- We acknowledge that any sense of injury or trauma for you [mother or birthing person] is important.[24]

Sheena Byrom has some interesting wisdom to share on this topic:

*'From time to time my colleagues would ask me, "does using different words really matter Sheena? We don't mean harm and what we do is more important than what we say. We have enough to worry about!" But my answer was (and is) it does matter. Because what we say and how we say it, influences what we do. If we are mindful of the language we use ( i.e.* facilitate *not* teach, share *instead of* educate*) we are thinking about the relationship we have with women and families and our actions will reflect that. Being with, not doing to. It doesn't take much effort, and needs no extra resources.'* [25]

 ## MOVE THE MIND: THE POWER OF NOT YET

*'Another piece of wisdom that I would share with newer midwives is something I often have to remind myself. The short statement is that "you don't have to believe everything you think". There will, I'm sure, be many occasions where negative thoughts will seem so loud in your mind. "I can't do it!", "I'll never get that job", "I was so bad at that skill/job". Whilst it may be the loudest thought, you don't have to believe it.'* Grace, midwife[26]

You've probably all heard of a growth mindset. It's become a bit of a buzzword in education and personal development work since Stanford professor Carol Dweck's book *Mindset* came out in 2006.[27] Her studies reveal how our mindset shapes our entire personality, dictates how we interpret success, failure and effort, as well as how we approach learning, sport, work and relationships. Two mindsets

– learned from our parents, teachers, work culture and the media we consume – are a fixed mindset, or a growth mindset. See www.ted.com/talks/carol_dweck_the_power_of_believing_that_you_can_improve (2014).

A fixed mindset assumes that personal qualities such as intelligence and personality are innate and unchangeable. If you have a fixed mindset, you feel you must constantly prove yourself. It encourages the question – do I have 'enough' to survive or go on succeeding? Or if I have a lot of intelligence and everyone tells me so, how on earth do I always live up to that? This heavier place of a fixed mindset is one where setbacks equal failures, and mistakes equal evidence of fixed fundamental stories about ourselves: 'I'm no good at maths/using my hands/academic work', 'I'm so clumsy', 'I'll never be able to…' and where the story around *not* getting the job or promotion is 'I'm actually not (innately) talented enough.' You can see how quickly this can spiral into an intolerable 'I'll never be good enough… best off quitting now'.

Stories of superhero talent can reinforce a fixed mindset. Most fictional superheroes have innate abilities beyond the ordinary. Captain Marvel did not, I assume, have to go through a helpful and normal and growth-promoting 'I cannot yet fly and shoot energy blasts from my hands but I'll keep practising' stage of life. It brings us back to the sharp question of where is the space *to* fail, learn and make more mistakes within a medical superhero narrative? One of the most poignant scenes in the final episode of *This is Going to Hurt* shows Erika, traumatised mother of a severely premature baby, giving Adam two 'World's Best Doctor' mugs, one for him and one for Shruti. He is called away to an emergency before he can explain that Shruti (boxed into the fear and recrimination of being World's Best Doctor, always having had to get it right – for her parents, for her community, difficult bosses, and patients) committed suicide the previous night.[28]

A growth mindset, on the other hand, always assumes that people can change and improve. If we choose to develop a growth mindset, we begin to believe the abilities we are born with are only a starting point – we can always learn more and shape ourselves with hard work, practice and experimentation. People with a growth mindset genuinely welcome mistakes as opportunities to learn, and challenges as a way to grow. As a starting point, it's way more playful and free, where instead of the statements in the left-hand column (and their echoes), we choose the ones on the right.

Which column are you more likely to land in? Circle the thoughts that most reflect your patterns. In which situations in the months ahead are you most likely to benefit from experimenting with trying out a growth mindset statement and the actions that may follow?

| Fixed mindset thoughts | Growth mindset thoughts |
| --- | --- |
| I'm useless at... | I'm not good at this right now... What am I missing? Who can support me? |
| I'm amazing at this | I'm on the right track |
| I give up | I'll try again with some of the strategies I've learned |
| This is too hard | This will take time and effort. Who can I reach out to for support? |
| I made a mistake. I feel ashamed and unworthy | Mistakes can be a gift – they can create honesty, humility, reflection and new learning |
| She's so brilliant. I will never be that competent/together/confident | I'm going to figure out how she does it and maybe even ask her. I'm going to remind myself to never compare someone else's external world with my internal world |

## MOVE THE MIND: THE POWER OF NOT TRUE

For years, I have held on to a story about being 'not practical'. It stems from some labelling as children – as the middle of three sisters I was the 'brainy, impractical' one, wrestling for space between the reliable one and the funny one – and has been reinforced with my 1980s education system-induced fixed mindset over the years and a burgeoning perfectionist streak bringing fear of trying and failing: 'I'm useless at DIY', 'I'm not much of a cook'. I had to face and be willing to let go of the old story as I went through midwifery training, to become a perfectly imperfect practical practising midwife and celebrate that we can all get better – at anything. In the grip of pressure or when (not if) I make a mistake, I can still find myself flooded with old storylines, one of which is 'I'm just not practical enough to do this job', but now I can catch it and see it for what it is.

Not true.

You might want to ask yourself these questions:

- What storylines have I been holding onto about myself and my capabilities that just aren't true anymore?
- Where could they shift?

Try this exercise, adapted from *How to Rise: A Complete Resilience Manual* by Chrissie Mowbray and Karen Forshaw.[29]

1. Cut or tear up some A4 paper into 24 pieces (more or less is fine).
2. On *each* small piece of paper write *one* role or label you have accepted over time. This might include traits and characteristics, and stories about yourself. Start with your name – maybe there were some expectations or stories that came even with the meaning behind your name? Then your gender. What comes with that? You are someone's child (write XXX's child) Are you a sibling? A parent? An aunt or uncle, niece or nephew? Are you someone's partner or lover? What are your 'titles' in the world? How does your current role in midwifery or maternity shape your identity? What roles or assumptions come from being someone's employee, team member or boss? What roles do you play during leisure time or within your family? Community organiser, Gatherer, Host, Carer, Shopper, Lynchpin? What other roles do you play in life? Feminist, Advocate, Speaker, Listener, for example? How might circumstances have given you unexpected roles – Patient, or

Victim for example? What characteristics have you accepted into your personality? Are you 'the funny one', 'the clever one', 'the organised one', 'the extrovert', 'the worrier'? How do others describe you? And how do you describe yourself?

3. Place another piece of A4 paper at the centre of the smaller pieces. This larger, central piece of paper represents you – in this moment as a blank page. Imagine all the roles, titles and labels sitting at the edges as connected to you, some by tiny fragile threads, and some as thick ropes, some by cords which are old and fraying. The strength and complexity of your attachment to those roles will shape what the ropes or threads look like. Use different coloured or width pens to sketch the cords if it helps to make the attachments visual. Remember that they are not actually who you are, just roles or labels that you have either chosen to pick up or that have become attached to you over time.

4. This is your chance to reimagine and release some cords. You will do this by bringing the roles that feel unequivocally 'you', true or wanted, directly onto the blank A4 sheet. Notice what you've included easily and what's still on the edge. Notice which roles you want to edge out further. When you look at those furthest out you can get excited. Try saying to yourself, 'I recognise the role that I have been playing up to now. It's not who I am, and it's not needed now, so I release my attachment to it.' Notice how it feels even to name what's true/not true/ needed/not needed any more. Either throw away the scrap of paper with that label on, or turn it over and on the blank side relabel it with something that feels true of you now. Take a photograph of the final paper with all the 'included' roles and stories. Discuss it with your trusted partner.

## MOVE THE MIND: ABCDEF FRAMEWORK FOR SHIFTING CORE BELIEFS AND FEELINGS

This is not an exercise as much as a framework to enable us to challenge our thoughts around any event by taking the additional powerful and necessary step of reframing our underlying core beliefs.

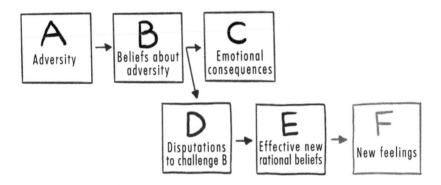

Albert Ellis developed a version of this model from its early form in the mid-1950s until his death in 2007 as part of his Rational Emotive Behaviour Therapy – the earliest form of what we now know as CBT or Cognitive Behavioural Therapy.[30]

It enables us to slow down enough (usually in reflection after an event) to see how easily we have leapt from the Activating event, or Adversity, to the Consequences – strong feelings, thoughts and actions – without examining the B: the Beliefs that are driving the big Cs. The slowing down not only reveals the self-defeating core Beliefs in the moment, but also invites us into D, Disputing those beliefs, E, choosing Effective new rational beliefs, and F, Feelings which are different to those possible to experience at A, B or C.

This is one to store in your back pocket, or even better as a series of headers in your journal, so that you can use it as a method of reflecting on any event that provokes strong feelings and beliefs in you. Practise working with your reflective group or trusted partner to use ABCDEF to reflect on the events and feelings you bring to each other.

| A – Activating Event | B – Beliefs (Dysfunctional) | C – Consequence |
|---|---|---|
| What has happened? What did I do? What did others do? What idea occurred to me? What emotions was I feeling? | What do I believe about the event? Which of my beliefs are my helpful/self-enhancing beliefs, and which are my dysfunctional/self-defeating beliefs? | Am I feeling anger, depression, anxiety, frustration, self-pity, etc? Am I behaving in a way that doesn't work for me (drinking, attacking, moping, etc)? |
| e.g. I didn't get the job that I wanted | e.g. I am worthless | e.g. I feel low about myself. I'm becoming demotivated and pulling away from the team |
| D – Dispute beliefs | E – Effective new belief | F - Feelings now |
| What is the evidence that my belief is true? In what ways is my belief helpful or unhelpful? | What helpful/self-enhancing new belief can I use to replace each self-defeating or dysfunctional belief? | What are my new feelings? |
| e.g. My colleagues and the families I work with see my worth. I have evidence in black and white in feedback. I'm going to gather that for my revalidation so I can see it all more clearly | e.g. I am good at my work most of the time but an interview is not my work. It requires a completely different set of skills and I need to prepare for those more thoroughly next time | e.g. I feel calmer and more motivated to take the action needed. I can look my team members in the eye and get on with the job before the next opportunity |

## MOVE THE MIND: TOOL FOR REFLECTION AND SELF-COMPASSION: RAIN ON YOUR THOUGHTS (TARA BRACH)

The acronym RAIN is an easy-to-remember practice and invitation in the midst of challenging feelings. **R**ecognise what is going on; **A**llow the experience to be there, just as it is; **I**nvestigate with interest and care; **N**urture with self-compassion.

You can take your time and explore RAIN as a stand-alone meditation at www.tarabrach.com/meditation-practice-rain or move gently through the steps whenever challenging feelings arise. Again, planting the acronym in your journal will help you return to it regularly via the visible reminder. Where the ABCDEF framework above is a very rational framework to alleviate the suffering created by dysfunctional core beliefs, RAIN relies primarily on the felt sense in our bodies to help experience the emotions more fully and leave space for readjustment. Different exercises or frameworks will appeal to different personality types and learning styles. Try them both on for size.

I have blended this exercise from two of Tara Brach's writings, using her own words to help further illuminate its gifts.[31]

### R – recognise what's going on

Recognising means consciously acknowledging, in any given moment, the thoughts, feelings, and behaviours that are affecting you. This can be a done with a simple mental whisper, noting what you are most aware of.

### A – allow the experience to be there, just as it is

Allowing means letting the thoughts, emotions, feelings, or sensations you have recognised simply be there, without trying to fix, avoid or change anything and without judging yourself for anything you are feeling.

You might recognise fear, and allow it by mentally whispering 'it's okay' or 'this belongs' or 'yes'.

Allowing creates a pause that makes it possible to deepen our attention.

### I – investigate with interest and care

To investigate, call on your natural curiosity... but stay in your body.

Many people initially see this word 'Investigate' as an invitation to fire up their cognitive skills – analysing the situation or themselves. But instead of thinking about what's going on, keep bringing your attention to your body, directly experiencing the sensations of vulnerability. Once you are fully present, listen for what this place truly needs.

You might ask yourself: what most wants attention? How am I experiencing this in my body? What is the most difficult/painful thing I am believing? What emotions does this bring up (fear, anger, grief)? Where are my feelings about this strongest in my body? When I assume the facial expression and body posture that best reflect these feelings and emotions, what do I notice? Are these feelings familiar, something I've experienced earlier in my life? If the most vulnerable, hurting part of me could communicate, what would it express (words, feelings, images)? What does this vulnerable place want from me? What does it most need?

Whatever the inquiry, your investigation will be most transformational if you step away from thinking and bring your primary attention to the felt-sense in the body.

## N – nurture with self-compassion

Self-compassion begins to naturally arise in the moments that you recognise you are suffering. It comes into fullness as you intentionally nurture your inner life with self-care.

To do this, try to sense what the wounded, frightened or hurting place inside you most needs, and then offer some gesture of active care that might address this need. Does it need a message of reassurance? Of forgiveness? Of companionship? Of love?

Experiment and see which intentional gesture of kindness most helps to comfort, soften or open your heart. It might be the mental whisper, I'm here with you. I'm sorry, and I love you. I love you, and I'm listening. It's not your fault.

In addition to a whispered message of care, many people find healing by gently placing a hand on the heart or cheek; or by envisioning being bathed in or embraced by warm, radiant light. If it feels difficult to offer yourself love, bring to mind a loving relationship – with God, family member, friend or pet – and imagine that being's love and wisdom flowing into you. You might choose to go there first and then, in the light and warmth of another's compassion, you may be able to offer self-compassion to yourself.

## After the RAIN

When you've completed the active steps of RAIN, it's important to notice the quality of your own presence and rest in that wakeful, tender space of awareness.

The fruit of RAIN is realising that you are no longer imprisoned in or identified with any limiting sense of self. What is life like when you don't believe the limiting thoughts? Who are you now in this moment?

Just notice… write or record that fruit if it helps capture the new story.

## MOVE THE MIND: THE BIG WORK/LIFE BALANCE DISTORTION – FINDING A NEW DEFINITION

Let's get it out there: I hate the phrase work/life balance.
How it sets work and 'life' in opposition, but also asks the impossible question of where will I find all those hours in the week to 'balance' the forty-odd I spend at work?

Instead, what would it be like to integrate work into a well-lived life?

From this perspective some different questions come to mind. You may find some fun overlap with the values playground exercise on p.148 and the ideal week exercise in ministering to the body as a discipline – what's in my week on p.167? If not, go back to them and try this in tandem.

Some different questions for you:

- To what extent am I wholeheartedly engaged in my life, including what I do at work?
- Am I bringing all of myself to family, friends, community, and my work, irrespective of how much time I spend in each of these areas?
- What do I value?
- To what extent does how I spend my time align with what I value?

- What do my team or colleagues value, and what can I do to support them in wholeheartedly engaging in their lives, including the work we do together?
- What might I want to change?

# CHAPTER 15

# IN THE WORKPLACE

*'If I could go back in time and talk to myself as a hopeful new midwife who thought she could change the world if she just sacrificed herself in the process, I'd remind her that doing so is not noble or necessary and that martyrdom only leads to misery further down the line. I'd remind her that setting and maintaining healthy boundaries and a work-life balance is crucial to thriving in any environment but especially in a profession as emotionally and physically taxing as midwifery. I'd remind her that in serving others, she mustn't stop serving herself, and that putting her own needs first is not selfish, it's sensible.'* Amity Reed, midwife[1]

So we move from the whole of life into the workplace, with more exercises to help us manage the daily challenges and bring the self-awareness and action that Amity is talking about into our midwifery lives. Brené Brown talks from her research of the dangerous ways we tend to self-protect at work: we choose 'certainty over curiosity, armour over vulnerability and knowing over learning'. She goes on to warn, 'shutting down comes with a price'[2] to our emotional and physical health, our creativity and ability to be fully with others. Move the body, move the breath, move the mind are *all the more applicable* here. Practice by practice they help us remain more open, more agile, more aware.

I'd like to highlight again that we are *not* talking here about wishy-washy side-stepping of real issues.

I love what Agnes Otzelberger, humanitarian aid worker, now researcher into compassion fatigue, says about the conflict resolution practice Just Like Me you will find below in the Move the mind section:

*'This practice is not about denying disagreement, violence or injustice. It is critical that we do give ourselves the space and*

*permission to feel the anger, bewilderment, rage or whatever*
*challenging emotions that come up in us. I say this because*
*practices like [this] are so often misunderstood as "pacifiers"*
*intended to make us apathetic towards injustice and suffering (and*
*are indeed often misused in that way). This is where grounding*
*the practice in a clear intention comes in: it can help us avoid this*
*trap of wanting to bypass difficulty and escape into some kind*
*of superficial bliss that disconnects us even further from what is*
*happening.'*[3]

## MOVE THE BODY: LOOK UP

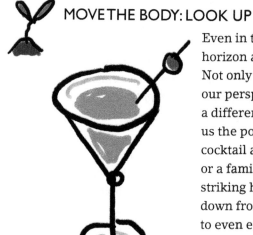

Even in the absence of a window and a
horizon at work, raising our gaze has benefits.
Not only does consciously looking up change
our perspective momentarily, but it also uses
a different part of the visual brain, and gives
us the potential to release a delicious chemical
cocktail as we smile or say hi to a colleague
or a family. This may sound obvious, but it is
striking how easily we can go head down-shut
down from each other when it feels too busy
to even engage with the risk that we might
be asked to stretch ourselves further. A lot of
midwifery work, particularly documentation
and medicines management, is also precise
and detailed. A lifted gaze into the middle distance or just above
the 'horizon' pulls our eye muscles against gravity and habit and
expands the periphery of our visual field, opening up possibilities or
connection with others. Eyes to the sky or even to the fluorescent lit
ceiling tiles (especially when accompanied by a personal faith) can
bring the helpful perspective that in this tiny corner of this indistinct
ward on an average Tuesday night, we are part of a beautiful bigger
picture.

## MOVE THE BODY: 120-SECOND BODY AWARENESS WITH MIDWIFE HEART RATE AND HYDRATION

As midwives we are skilled at 'reading the room', using our senses to pick up shifts in mood, need or physiology. This exercise invites us to use those same senses to observe what is happening in our own bodies, taking stock and redressing imbalances, just as we are doing for the women and families we care for. You could choose an hourly review in a labour room or walking to collect the next pregnant woman after three compressed clinic appointments. The aim is to return you to your body for 60 seconds and then act on what you find. As Sheena Byrom wisely says 'Midwives, listen to your own and the mother's heart, as well as the baby's'.[4]

- Place two fingers on your own pulse and take 60 seconds to breathe deeply and consciously. Use the square breath or *ujayi* breath (see pp.174-175) if you like them.
- As you do, notice your dry mouth, and any sensations in your head, scan down your body, focusing particularly on releasing tightness and tension in your chest and belly.
- Take the next 60 seconds to drink 500ml of water, unapologetically. You are quite literally topping up your own resources before you can meet the needs of this person.
- As you settle back into your next task or conversation, think, what needs to change for me, emotionally or positionally?
- Finally, think what request could I make (from this client 'please bring a urine sample ready from home next time', from a senior midwife 'I need an early lunch today if possible', from a colleague 'could you send my bloods with yours?') that would be a stress reducer for you today?

## MOVE THE BODY: 120-SECOND TENSION RELEASE

Tension releasing stretches make such a difference to our long work days, especially after the leaning, lifting, hunching, steering (wayward beds and wheelchairs and cars!) we do as midwives. We also spend hours typing or writing notes in less than optimal conditions. The earlier we are able to identify signs of tension and stress, the quicker we can use these exercises to take action. The most helpful way to use stretches is to find a sequence that works for you, or that directly addresses your vulnerable spots as well as where you tend to hold tension. Interestingly, when you search the trusty web for 'stretches for midwives' or 'midwives' body awareness' you get one hardy Australian blog drowned out by yoga for pregnancy and wellbeing for mums. This says a lot about how midwives' bodies have been deprioritised in service of birthing women. While this is understandable, it is also something we need to resist.

Many trusts have a physiotherapist within their wellbeing team, who while distant to most of us might be able to help create a quick and easy sequence. That helps with accountability. If someone's going to check in on us and ask 'How's it going? How are you doing preserving your physical integrity in this crazy job?' we are more likely to do the stretches. Others doing them helps too, so decide together with a few colleagues that this is going to be part of your next few shifts and compare notes. The other thing we can do is ask ourselves 'How else can I set myself up for success?' That might be 'orientating' the couple in a labour room to the fact that you might do some stretches every hour and that they are welcome to join in. It cues you all up for using some biomechanics in the room too, as it sets the expectation of using movement to correct, release and restore.

Try something in a sequence of your choice: side to side neck turns or tilts, gentle chin to chest stretches, shoulder shrugs, chest opening with hands interlocked behind back, wrist rotations, hip lifts or rotations, calf stretches, ankle rotations, rocking onto tiptoes.

## MOVE THE BODY: FIVE-FINGER EXERCISE

This is a lovely quick and effective exercise adapted from David Cheek,[5] bringing a lift to both mood and sense of self. It is a powerful way to make you smile as you start a break, opening a gateway to endorphins and oxytocin, or to reset when moving from a challenging situation into a completely different context or family.

*Touch your thumb to your index finger with a deep breath... As you do this, remember a time when your body felt healthy fatigue... Perhaps you* had just engaged in an exhilarating physical activity. Feel it now in your muscles...

Touch your thumb to your middle finger with a deep breath... As you do so, go back to a time when you had a loving experience. It may be sexual... It may be a warm embrace... Or an intimate conversation. Access as many senses as you can as you recall that moment: smell, sound, touch, taste as well as sight.

Touch your thumb to your ring finger with a deep breath... As you do so, go back to the best acknowledgement you have ever received. Try to receive it more deeply in this moment. By welcoming it and believing it, you are also honouring the person who said it. Picture him or her now as you let the truth of that acknowledgement seep into your body...

Touch your thumb to your little finger with a deep breath... As you do so, go back to the most beautiful place you have ever been. Stay there for a while, taking in the colours and scents – the beauty of that place.

## MOVE THE BODY: FEET ON THE FLOOR GROUNDING STRATEGY (see also tree visualisation on p.172)

This is an incredibly helpful exercise to do in a couple of minutes in preparation for or even in the midst of a stressful event or a difficult conversation. It is possible to do it in a chair, anchoring into that moment using your feet, but this version has you standing. It can even be done mindfully on the way to the loo.

Feet on the Floor: Grounding Strategy with Diana Tikasz (available at www.tendacademy.ca/feet-on-the-floor/)

Start with a soft gaze or your eyes closed, then move your awareness: focus into the soles of your feet, placing your full attention there. Notice in your feet the points of contact with the floor. Notice the distribution of weight. Gently rolling your feet back and forth, notice the changes in sensation in the feet, changes in distribution of weight. Moving from side to side. Notice the subtle small changes... When your mind wanders off... that's okay. When you notice it, bring your attention back to the soles of your feet, anchoring to the floor. Walk very slowly. What happens to the sensations when you lift one foot and place it on the floor, noticing the distribution of weight? You may want to take one step back and see how *that feels. You may notice how small the surface area of the feet is. You may feel some gratitude for your feet and all the work they do all day to keep you upright. When you are ready, release the focus on the soles of your feet. Notice how your whole body feels now as you raise your eyes and return to the task or conversation ahead.*

## MOVE THE BREATH: SQUEEGEE BREATH – THREE-SECOND RECOVERY

Any of the breath practices from the previous chapter: change breath, balancing breath, square breath, ujayi breath are gifts: quickly deployed and very effective at enabling us to find our centre at work. Here's one more.

*After a relentless clinic or an intense experience on the wards, our level of awareness in that moment is a bit like a dirty window. We can use our breath and our mind to clean it.*

*Set your intention for where you want to be next: fully present in a meeting, listening to the next woman in an antenatal appointment, simply sitting and eating lunch.*

*Take a deep breath all the way to the top of your head. Count 1,2,3. Breathe out and imagine that squeegee going all the way down your body, all the way to the bottom of your toes. You have released everything that doesn't need to be there. Breathe. And you're present. Breathe. And smile.*

## MOVE THE MIND: TINY HABITS

With all of these quick breath or many other practices, we get to choose to integrate them into our work lives as tiny habits. Tiny habits is an approach developed by B.J. Fogg of the Behaviour Design Lab at Stanford University. [6] Focusing on really tiny actions (or starter actions which are just a tiny part of the action) that we can do in less than thirty seconds, the idea is that we can fit them naturally into life by linking them to regular/automatic anchor moments like walking out to collect the next family in clinic, brushing teeth, washing hands, the first 30 seconds in the car before driving home. You then link it to a tiny celebration. The theory goes that when something is tiny, it's easy to do – which means you don't need to rely on the unreliable nature of motivation. The key is to scale it back to something *really* simple like:

- after I brush my teeth I will floss one tooth
- after I walk into the kitchen I will get a lemon out of the fridge
- after I drink water on shift I will take one squeegee breath
- after I get into the car to drive home I will hold on to the car key in the ignition (starter action) until I've said out loud, 'Despite everything, today I'm proud that I...'. The key here is you don't even need to plan to finish the sentence. It's just the starting itself that begins to work the habit into life, and the celebration that follows helps to create a dopamine hit that begins to wire the brain to want to do it again.

B.J. Fogg calls the celebration:

*'habit fertilizer... each individual celebration strengthens the roots of a specific habit, but the accumulation of celebrations over time is what fertilizes the entire habit garden. By cultivating feelings of success and confidence, we also make the soil more inviting and nourishing for all the other habit seeds we want to plant.'*[7]

A celebration could be a smile, a deep nourishing breath, a moment of just saying 'yes!' or 'well done me'. All of these things reshape our brain chemistry to experience reward.

Try out the Tiny Habits recipe:

- After I (regular, every day moment)...
- I will (really small thing that you don't need to think about but will just do)...
- Then I will (celebration)...

## MOVE THE MIND: RITUALS OF TRANSITION – HOME TO WORK/WORK TO HOME

Tiny habits are like mini rituals. Even if we live a very varied life, we all rely on rituals through our day to help with a feeling of stability and comfort. Transition rituals might include deliberately changing clothes, mindfully putting clothes 'away', like a packing away of the day, taking 10 minutes if possible to shift gears in a place that you love, like a park, integrated into your commute if possible. In their study of resilient midwives Billie Hunter and Lucie Warren heard midwives describing their effective journey rituals of shifting gears, gaining perspective and reflecting:

> 'What helps me is getting on the bus and the train after the shift and watching other people in their lives with their conversations and just emptying my brain or slowly pondering an event at work...'[8]

One way to make the transition is to try this unpacking ritual:

### Unpacking the bag – choosing what's welcome and what's not

*Picture yourself leaving work with a full bag, stuffed full of feelings, memories, other people's emotions as well as your own. One or two of them are welcome, and you can carry them into your home. Others have snuck their way into your bag and you'd rather leave them aside before you get home.*

*Whether you are driving, walking or on the bus, bring your attention to your breath. Notice the sensation of coming back into your body and feeling your breath again after the busiest last few hours. Picture the bag full of objects you have walked out with. In your imagination, take out the one you are happy to keep or take home with you. Feel it in your hands. What does it feel like? What positive moment does it represent? Place it right at the bottom of your bag. It will remain there and be available to you when your housemate or partner says 'How was your day?'*

*Now turn your attention to the other objects on top, the ones you want to leave behind. Take out the first. Again notice what it feels like in your hands, notice the colour, the texture of this object, the temperature, the weight. Notice what feeling, person or situation it represents. Now observe it getting lighter and lighter in your hands until it begins to hover and float. Use your breath to physically blow it away (like a bubble). As you blow and it moves away, try out saying to yourself 'I*

*honour the importance of this person/situation/feeling by choosing*
*distance and rest'. It has not disappeared completely, just been carried*
*on the wind. You can return to it when you need to. And in the meantime*
*you have chosen distance and rest. Repeat this process with the*
*remaining unwelcome items in the bag until the only thing remaining is*
*the welcome item, visible and accessible should you choose to bring it*
*out when you get home.*

### Repacking the bag – reclaiming energy

You could use this one at any point in your day when you feel like
your energy is depleted or when a sense of powerlessness has crept
in. It also works for a journey home when you are physically and
emotionally depleted. The focus is reclaiming your energy whenever
you need to.

*Wherever you are, bring your awareness to your breathing, noticing*
*the flow in and out. As you continue to focus, let those breaths slow and*
*deepen and let the out-breath each time be a moment when you release*
*a little more tension, a little more deeply. Notice, where does your feeling*
*of exhaustion or depletion show up in your body? What's the sensation?*
*Does it have a colour? A taste? A smell? Just sit or walk with that*
*sensation for a minute.*

*Now picture a path – a journey ahead. If you are walking, you can use*
*the actual path in front of you. This is the path where you can reclaim*
*your energy. Start walking either in reality or in your mind's eye. As you*
*walk, you can see objects left along the edges, which represent the energy*
*you have lost or given away today. It doesn't matter what they are exactly,*
*although you might decide to notice that. The important thing is that as you*
*walk you can pick up these objects and put them in your bag, which starts*
*empty and begins to fill. Go on collecting the lost objects, until you reach*
*the end of the journey. You'll know when this is. Now imagine sitting down*
*with your bag in a place where you can look inside. The contents have*
*become a ball of colour, which is yours. Take it out and breathe this moving*
*colour energy into your chest, or hold it close. Enjoy the sensation of filling*
*with dynamic colour as you receive and absorb your energy again. As you*
*slowly come back to fuller awareness of the world around you, notice what*
*it feels like in your body to be replenished and ready for your next step.*

## MOVE THE MIND: SELF-CARE TRAFFIC LIGHT EARLY-WARNING SYSTEM

Françoise Mathieu, in her *Compassion Fatigue Workbook*,[9] suggests we imagine a green, amber, red style dosimeter, like the ones radiologists wear to warn them of over-exposure. We usually know when our built-in warning system is flagging signs of stress. I get tight in my neck and shoulders, sometimes in my jaw. Colleagues of mine feel a migraine coming on. Can we identify our other warning signs of exposure to trauma? How does trauma exposure or compassion fatigue begin to show up in me? See p.80 for the 16 signs of trauma exposure response.

Imagine 'plugging in' your dosimeter as you leave work. Is it reading green, amber or red?

Ask yourself

- What signs and symptoms do I bring home with me most often?
- What signs and symptoms did I experience at work today?
- What is it costing me to live like this?
- What one small step can I take tomorrow/now to bring down my 'toxin' levels?
- Who can help me with this?

## MOVE THE MIND: KNOWING YOUR WINDOW OF TOLERANCE

The 'window of tolerance' is a term coined by Dr Dan Siegel.[10,11] It is used to describe normal reactions in the brain and body, especially following challenging situations. The idea is that within our optimal arousal level we can tolerate or manage the ups and downs of human life. We may experience emotions such as hurt, anxiety, pain and anger that move us to the upper borders of the window of tolerance, or there may be times when we are so exhausted, sad or shut down that we touch on the lower borders, but most of us have self-regulation strategies – developed out of co-regulation strategies we learned with our caregivers – that help us stay within the window. The dotted line in the diagram below shows the natural ebb and flow of a nervous system which is regulating itself. When we experience trauma, our nervous systems can be profoundly disrupted. Our senses are heightened, our reactions are more intense. We are less likely to be able to access conscious or even unconscious strategies to regulate ourselves. We are more likely in this state of stress to get thrown off balance. Also our window of tolerance shrinks in the wake of adverse experiences – and those with childhood trauma already have a narrower window of tolerance – so we have less scope, less space to ebb and flow and a greater tendency to become overwhelmed and move into either hyper or hypo arousal. The solid more jagged line in the diagram is a dysregulated response, moving

### sharply into hyperarousal

Which involves excessive activation, often in the form of anxiety, panic, fear, hypervigilance, emotional flooding. Our nervous system is stuck without an off switch, affecting our ability to sleep, eat and digest and manage our emotions.

### then into hypoarousal

Which can happen as a result of excessive, unmanageable hyperarousal. This is a state of shutting down or dissociating. Our nervous system here has lost the 'on' button and we might experience exhaustion, depression, numbness and disconnection.

Neither hyperarousal nor hypoarousal are usually something we choose. The reaction just takes over. The body wants to either move into a persistent fight/flight state, or into freeze.

We saw in Part I (p.75) that research has shown that trauma exposure can shift us into a state of hypoarousal such that only hyperarousal moments (such as in the emergency moment) make us feel truly alive.[12,13] This is obviously a distortion, bypassing the optimal arousal zone completely.

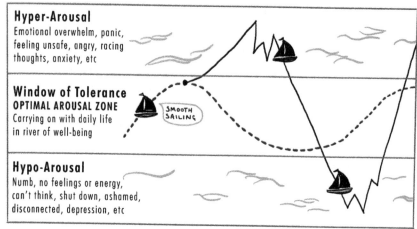

**Hyper-Arousal**
Emotional overwhelm, panic, feeling unsafe, angry, racing thoughts, anxiety, etc

**Window of Tolerance**
**OPTIMAL AROUSAL ZONE**
Carrying on with daily life in river of well-being

SMOOTH SAILING

**Hypo-Arousal**
Numb, no feelings or energy, can't think, shut down, ashamed, disconnected, depression, etc

Image: St. Michael's Hospital, Toronto, ON. Mindful Awareness Stabilization Training (MAST)

The good news for those of us exposed to stress and trauma in our work is that we can work with our window of tolerance by exploring what happens to us when we move into the borderlands.

Answer these questions on your own, with your group or your trusted partner:

- What are the big three warning signs I experience – eye twitch, irritable bowel, back pain, headache, stomach acid – when I am moving out of my window? How is my body letting me know and how am I responding to it? (see also Part I, p.80 for 16 signs of trauma exposure response).
- What is my number one behaviour when heading into hyperarousal?
- What are some of the emotional reactions I have?

## MOVE THE MIND: LOW-IMPACT DEBRIEFING – STRATEGIES TO AVOID (RE)TRAUMATISING OTHERS

Traumatising others with our stories is so easy to do unknowingly. It's eye-opening to consider that practising story stewardship is not just about protecting confidentiality, but also knowing that the story has value – to the people involved of course, but also to the casual listener. The story may have the potential to harm.

Françoise Mathieu, author of the *Compassion Fatigue Workbook* and founder of the TEND academy, suggests we think of the traumatic stories we witness and hear in our work as being contained behind a tap – allowing us to decide how much we release, and at what pace.[14] She suggests we:

### Increase self-awareness
By deliberately auditing one or two weeks at work and recording how, where, and in what way we have been debriefing difficult stories. Also notice (as you will still be close to the time when it happened) what was actually helpful, and what wasn't.

### Think about the setting and expectations of that setting
Is it a catch-up in the car park, a Christmas party, a formal debrief, a casual chat on labour ward?

### Give fair warning
Just as we would not deliver bad news to a family without fair warning in the form of 'I have some bad news' or 'Let's sit down', a warning gives the listener an opportunity to mentally prepare for what you are about to say.

### Get consent
You might say 'I heard something really terrible. Is it okay if I talk to you about it?' This gives the listener the opportunity to say no, or to clarify what the subject matter is and whether they are the right person to hear it.

### Choose to limit your disclosure
Mathieu suggests imagining starting on the outer circle of the story (the least traumatic information) and slowly moving in toward the core. At each stage, you get to decide. Do I need to go further or not? Do I have consent to go further? Is the listener able to control the flow in any way?[15]

Experiment with using this low-impact debriefing. Notice how different it feels when you have consent, or when you actively control the flow. Do you feel debriefed? If you're interested in this, discuss setting up a session for you and your colleagues about low-impact debriefing with your PMA, if you're in England, or another suitable person.

## MOVE THE MIND: A REVOLUTIONARY APPROACH TO STRENGTHS

What's it like for you at work not to be 'seen' for all of who you are and what you can offer? Are you one of the midwives who, at one time or another, has asked to stay in a favourite area of midwifery and been told you really need to be able to maintain skills everywhere? Of course, there are certain basic things we all need to be able to do safely as midwives. Yet a truly flourishing organisation will enable people to work where they feel most able to use and grow their distinctive qualities. We've all had appraisals or PDRs where the emphasis has been on 'improving' on weaker areas. That's the conventional way of seeing growth, as roundedness. 'Playing to our strengths', on the other hand, has almost become a cliché. What a relief then to prepare for your next key conversation with this refreshing tool which enables you to recognise and:

- name and moderate your learned behaviours (Yes, I'm good at that and everyone knows it, but it actually *drains* me)
- claim and marshall your realised strengths (Yes! I'm good at that, I'm using it and it energises me)

and finally, here's the rub:

- dare to go to the max with unrealised strengths (Vroom! Yes indeed I'm good at them, they energise me, I'm not using them much)
- laugh at your weaknesses (Ha ha! All is well. What if someone else – who loves doing that! – could do it?....

For example, I have a colleague who genuinely gets a kick out of the speedy processing of computer discharges on the postnatal ward, and is happy to measure the success of her day by how many people she can move on and how quickly. Great! I'll happily do them, but not as quickly as her and definitely not with so much joy. When I get to the end of the shift I won't be counting discharges as a measure of a good day. On the other hand, I love having those conversations which despatch a new family into the outside world with more confidence and a renewed perspective on their new phase of life. I can do that efficiently but also tenderly and with genuine compassion for what they are about to encounter. Great! We are both on postnatal ward that day, but let's discuss dividing the tasks so that we play to our strengths. How much more satisfaction might we find if we got to design our place of work choices around this (plus values, purpose and everything you have explored in Chapter 13)?

We can't all be brilliant at everything. What a relief! That's why we have each other.

Working it out in a trusted pair:

Try sitting down with a colleague who really knows you and working out together what you would put in each of these boxes. Be really honest with each other.

| UNREALISED STRENGTHS | REALISED STRENGTHS |
|---|---|
| I'm good at them. They energise me. I'm not using them. | I'm good at them. They energise me. I'm using them. |
| RELATIVE WEAKNESSES | LEARNED BEHAVIOURS |
| I'm not good at them. | I'm good at them. They drain me. |

## MOVE THE MIND: EXERCISES FOR MINIMISING THE IMPACT OF CONFLICT

When we encounter an 'other' person whose behaviours violate our values or sense of safety, there are ways in which we can minimise the impact. Tara Brach's RAIN on p.189 is a useful practice here just to observe closely what we are feeling. Here are two more.

## MOVE THE MIND (CONFLICT): CLOAK OF PROTECTION

One of the features of the environments we work in is that we are often exposed to others' strong feelings of frustration, urgency, panic, anger, vulnerability, pain or grief – from both colleagues and families. A wise colleague of mine once talked about her strategy for walking on to labour ward and it stuck.

> 'I just put on my cloak and it means any words or arrows coming my way can slide off rather than stick to me or wound me.'

The cloak – a powerful historical image of protection, with texture, weight and gravitas – can indeed prevent us from absorbing others' emotions or protect us from being triggered, especially when our window of tolerance (see p.202) is narrowed by events.

The exercise below is brief. A longer seven-minute version can be found here, voiced by the legendary nurse and academic, person-centred care pioneer Brendan McCormack: www.youtube.com/watch?v=drGA50RMJ7Y

*Begin by bringing your attention to your breathing, just watching the breath as it is. Then start slowing and deepening those breaths, taking the air right down into the bottom of your lungs. Begin to allow the out-breath to become just a little bit longer than the in breath... As you gently deepen and lengthen that out-breath, begin to let go of any tension that you have been holding in your body. Soften your tongue in your mouth. Touch the tip of your tongue to just behind your front teeth and let it rest. Soften your jaw and then your belly. As your body softens on the inside, choose to place a soft cloak around your outside – a cloak that can protect you from words or emotions that don't belong to you. Feel the warmth and texture of the cloak. What's it like to be in it? What do you notice most about the experience of wearing it? As you breathe, notice that wrapped in the cloak, you can be the observer, a wise, even version of yourself. From here you get to see situations calmly, as they actually are. And time feels different when you wear the cloak. There is more space between words and between thoughts. You can hear the silences and pauses – not just the words. You can see the bigger picture – and choose how to respond. Breathe now and know that you can access your cloak at any time.*

## MOVE THE MIND (CONFLICT): JUST LIKE ME (BY JOEL AND MICHELLE LEVEY)

This exercise can be done in pairs, by two people facing each other (one representing the 'other' involved in the conflict), or alone, by bringing to mind the person who you are finding difficult to be with. It can be done silently, when meeting someone new and confronted by a clash of values or feelings. You can use any or all of these phrases, or any that seem appropriate. It's amazing how difficult emotions can shift and new conversations can open up even when this is done just with the person 'pictured' in front of you. In other words, because we are part of any system, when our perspective shifts, the system shifts with it.

Try it out:

*Become aware that there is a person in front of you – in reality, or in your imagination. A fellow human being, just like you.*
*Now silently repeat these phrases, while looking at them.*

*This person has a body and a mind, just like me.*
*This person has feelings, emotions and thoughts, just like me.*
*This person has in his or her life, experienced physical and emotional pain and suffering, just like me.*
*This person has at some point been sad, disappointed, angry, or hurt, just like me.*
*This person has felt unworthy or inadequate, just like me.*
*This person worries and is frightened sometimes, just like me.*
*This person has longed for friendship, just like me.*

*This person is learning about life, just like me.*
*This person wants to be caring and kind to others, just like me.*
*This person wants to be content with what life has given, just like me.*
*This person wishes to be free from pain and suffering, just like me.*
*This person wishes to be safe and healthy, just like me.*
*This person wishes to be happy, just like me.*
*This person wishes to be loved, just like me.*

*Now, allow some wishes for well-being to arise:*

*I wish that this person have the strength, resources, and social support to navigate the difficulties in life with ease.*
*I wish that this person be free from pain and suffering.*
*I wish that this person be peaceful and happy.*
*I wish that this person be loved.*
*Because this person is a fellow human being, just like me.*

*After a few moments, thank the person in whatever way feels appropriate.*

## MOVE THE MIND (CONFLICT): MY SHAME STORY

When our vulnerabilities meet others' vulnerabilities, conflict can easily arise. You have already done some digging into your story, motivations and purpose. This exercise will enable you to see how your vulnerabilities might be playing their part.

To come right to the heart of this, let's talk about shame. Shame is one of the hugely under-researched areas that Brené Brown has been uncovering in her work. When shame is present, we are saying not just 'I have done wrong', but 'I am wrong. I am unworthy of love, connection or belonging'. One of the main ways in which shame casts its shadow is when we 'fail' to meet the impossible and often contradictory expectations of society or of others. So it shows up all the time, especially in clinical settings, when the expectation is that we are able to eliminate both risk and mistakes, not to mention go on fulfilling the superhero narrative without the internal or external resources to do so. Shame is a strong sensation often felt viscerally in our body first, with a dry mouth, heart racing, time slowing down and so on.

Certain roles such as mothering (and midwifing) suffer from particularly high and particularly contradictory expectations. Every time we inadvertently reinforce them – on social media or otherwise – we together form what Brené Brown calls a 'shame web', which mostly makes us hide our shame in secrecy or silence. Shame can also make us judgemental towards others who show the very weaknesses that *we* feel shame about – a massive recipe for conflict. Brown's research sees these weaknesses relating to an 'unwanted identity': a type of person we cannot bear to be seen as; we distance ourselves from that identity by judging and criticising anyone who seems to behave in that way.[16]

Try this powerful exercise adapted from Brené Brown:[17]

### What is my physical response to shame?

*How do I know when it's coming?*

*When I feel shame I feel...*

### What are my shame triggers?

I suffered from being trapped in the silent shame web around motherhood in the very early years, wanting to live up to an ideal of being a calm, present and creative mother while juggling it all effortlessly with my career. I also had a completely contradictory ideal of being a mother with a tidy home, instilled deep in me as a consequence of shame and judgement from my own mother about mess. In truth, much of the time I was overwhelmed by the chaos of family life, pulling in and out emotionally, too tired to think, let alone be creative. Writing down these wanted and unwanted identities, as you are about to, helps me understand how my and others' perceptions make me more vulnerable to shame. Try it now:

Pick *one* shame category (your body, your work, addiction, money, motherhood, parenting etc).

Name it.

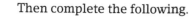

Then complete the following.

*Write down 3–5 ideal identities*
I want to be perceived as…

*Write down 3–5 unwanted identities*
I do *not* want to be perceived as…

For *each* of your unwanted identities, answer these questions:

- What does this perception mean to me?
- Why is it so unwanted?
- Where did the messages that fuel this unwanted identity come from?

So I have an unwanted identity about being mediocre. In fact, on a coaching training course many years ago I spent the weekend wearing a badge saying 'mediocre' to help increase my ability to 'be with it'. For me it comes from being the middle of three girls in quick sibling succession – an easy place to get lost, and getting stuck in perceiving 'perfect' to be the most attention or affection-grabbing outcome as a child. Mediocre sets off a primal panic in me, and triggers judgement of myself and others. Perfect of course is completely unattainable, and creates the stage for shame's disco party.

You will be able to see from *your* answers that shame is likely active in your life, setting off chemical reactions with the experiences or vulnerabilities that you brought into this work. Perhaps it was one of your unwanted identities (possibly linked to trauma exposure, which is common in those in the helper professions) that became the driver for you getting into this work in the first place? Next time you are in a moment of conflict with a colleague, a family member or your partner, notice how your wanted and unwanted identities might be playing their part. Speak to your trusted partner or journal about what you are discovering.

# CHAPTER 16

# SMALL CHANGE, BIG IMPACT: HOW TO ENGAGE IN CHANGE

*'I do know that I am a product of a rich and deep culture, which makes me unique in the way that I practice. My experiences, upbringing and heritage as part of a Black family and community are tools that I can incorporate into my passion to provide care. Whilst it sometimes feels like all practitioners should be the same, sound the same and operate in the same way, I know that I, and indeed all of us have a varied set of skills, which we use to approach scenarios in very different ways.'* Grace, midwife[1]

Look back to the exercise 'My voice as an instrument' on p.150.

Your voice is just one part of you, but as we start to think about you as a change-maker, this is a reminder of what you bring. Every part of you brings something distinctive to the conversation.

## WHY BE A CHANGE-MAKER?

One of the inevitable impacts of burnout and trauma exposure that we discussed in Part I is a distancing from work and the kind of engagement needed to work on new ways forward. It's completely understandable, therefore, that you might feel like running a mile from being a 'change-maker'. And I get it – you are also tired. And worried that you might not get the buy-in you need to go ahead.

Allow me just to put the case for tiny change in the form of a small, distinct project that you really care about, in the company of colleagues or families who also care.

Taking action stokes hope. And hope brings with it the perspective that small change can make a big impact.[2]

Doctors Wendy Dean and Simon Talbot are doing more than anyone else in the world at the moment to raise the profile of the impact of moral injury. They say:

> 'In order to make real change, we will need to engage "activists" from all aspects of the health care system – clinicians, health care administrators, policymakers, and, above all, patients and their families – to pitch in to address the structural causes of moral injury in health care.'[3]

In other words, in order to address moral injury, we will need to recruit those who are suffering from its effects. A major challenge, but research shows that taking action, in the form of small steps, is healing in itself. This makes sense as in taking action we get to realign with our values and purpose, we feel more integrated, and less isolated and 'distant' as we build community around us to effect our tiny change.

Research involving midwives directly has also highlighted the power of proactivity and self-efficacy as a building block of longevity and satisfaction in midwifery. The sense of autonomy and measure of control that a small project can bring is also significant.[4,5]

## WHAT COULD YOU DO?

Look back to the exercises on recalling the midwifery dream, your purpose and in particular your Big Why. The one where you said 'I want to live in a world where... because it's not okay that... so I'm going to...'. What bugs you most? What do you long to see change?

Here's a selection of small but significant changes I've already mentioned in Part I. Notice as you read them whether you are drawn to any.

- Reimagining the handover
- Reimagining the midwife's role at caesarean birth
- Reimagining space to reflect
- Reimagining how conversations about hard things happen
- Reimagining the healthy and consistent response to an adverse event

- Reimagining midwives' involvement in designing the rota

Perhaps your tiny project relates to a part of the current process:

- Reimagining the booking appointment
- Reimagining the 'discharge' conversation

Or to a particular group:

- Reimagining our relationships with refugee women
- Reimagining our notes for trans/non-binary people
- Reimagining access to senior roles for Black, Brown and Mixed Ethnicity staff

If time/money/energy were no object, what would you do? Write it down.

A caveat here: what follows is a brief Small Change 101, deserving a whole volume, but intentionally planting tools and resources (see Resources Home section) in your hands to get started.

## MORE ON MINDSET

Choosing a mindset of 'there is enough' time/money/energy is profoundly counter-cultural, but a major step in initiating your tiny project. A scarcity mentality is often set deep into our lives – doctors in particular have grown up in a culture of having to compete for grades and fight for jobs. All striving, comparison and competitiveness comes, in part at least, from a sense of scarcity. The scarcity mentality is pervasive in the NHS, born originally out of an era of hardship. Even in times of plenty (of supplies and staff) this mindset persists, and most recently, of course, we've been hit by a pronounced staff scarcity. These are systemic issues, but they trickle down into our own mentality. They play out in small ways – cue rolling eyes, a mantra of 'never enough', cheap cups and warm watered dust masquerading as a cup of tea.

We also each have our own relationship to scarcity and abundance, influenced by the scripts of our early lives. I've been heavily influenced by a scarcity mindset because of how my father grew up. So I have to work every day to catch myself and replace the lie of 'not enough' with truth of 'plenty – just look around'. My Christian faith helps me to see this too. How might what I need be already here? What would resource-full look like on this project? Who or what might be part of this? You can see how the chosen perspective – of working from abundance – raises our motivation and agility to look for solutions in creative ways. This is not being naive –there will be obstacles which take energy and creativity to overcome (together). It gives us a helpful starting place.

### Be clear about your circle of control/influence

This is an exercise to do on your own and to repeat together with your tribe/tiny project team. It helps us see more clearly what we can and can't control, and those things that we can influence but not control. It also helps guide us to create a plan of action to tackle issues within our circle of influence – which can be harder to grasp.

Draw a large circle on an A4 sheet. Inside it draw two smaller circles.

The *circle of concern* is the outermost circle and it includes all areas you care about (most of which you probably can't do much about). Mark this outer ring with the activities or decisions relating to your tiny project over which you have no control.

The *circle of influence* is the middle ring, which contains the activities over which you have some control, but need others to help you. You will need to use your relationships and your communications to help you achieve this. It might take more time as a result. Our circle of influence has been compared to a muscle. It can expand and enlarge with exercise and get smaller with lack of use.

When we pay attention to the activities we can influence, for example via our relationships with colleagues, we can expand our knowledge and experience, and so the circle of influence increases. On the other hand, when we spend time and energy on the things we cannot control (in our circle of concern), like a decision over which we have no influence, or someone else's response to the tiny project idea, we have less time and energy to spend on things we can influence, so the circle of influence becomes smaller. Where we pay attention affects how we use our time and energy wisely.

Within the circle of influence is another circle – *the circle of control.* This is the smallest and innermost circle, representing those tasks and activities in the midst of your tiny project where you have control, or can action directly. Write down those areas or actions.

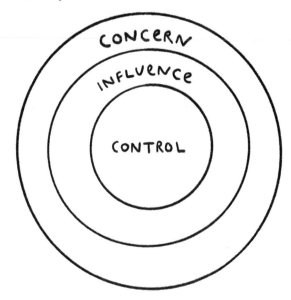

### Find your people

This is crucial. Going it alone (even with a tiny project) is hard. First look back to the exercise 'Finding your tribe – allies for the journey' on p.159 where you will find strategies for finding those internally and externally wanting or working on similar tiny change. It can take courage to approach the Director of Midwifery, consultant midwife or one of the obstetricians who you know is interested in the area of your tiny project. But remember that they would hate to think that it took courage to approach them. In their best moments they would relish opportunities to talk directly to midwives on the ground, especially those approaching them to ask for their backing for a tiny change.

Get together with your tribe and map out a together exercise: 'Together we will...', 'Together we believe', 'We want to live in a world where...'. The more imaginative you are, the more you will draw people in.

- Decide on how you want to communicate your vision to others.
- Include a wide range of other staff (outside of your core) early in the process so that you are using their words and wisdom.

### Use Appreciative Inquiry

Whoever you are engaging from the outset, Appreciative Inquiry is an approach which focuses us first on what we already do well in our tiny project area. It asks the fundamental question – what gives 'life' (...to the handover, to the theatre environment, to the booking appointment, to the recruitment process)? It explores strengths and past successes, aiming to understand what has enabled them. It's a useful way to shift current mindsets and vocabulary away from deficit/problem-focused thinking.[6]

These good news stories are then used to shape new possibilities that bridge the best of 'what is' with collective thinking on 'what might be', challenging the status quo and common assumptions about 'how things work around here'. Participants then use their individual strengths and combined insights to co-design a solution. So start with 'what works' in what currently exists.

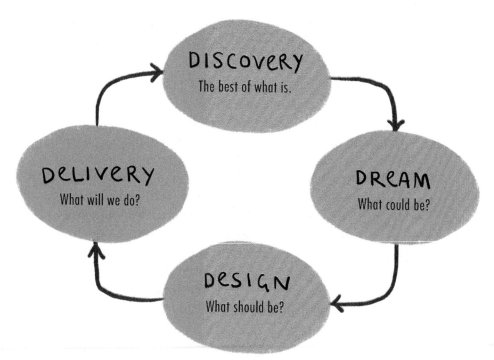

DISCOVERY
The best of what is.

DREAM
What could be?

DESIGN
What should be?

DELIVERY
What will we do?

## Acknowledge what or who has gone before

Even when systems are less than ideal, a tiny change (with a big impact), is always possible. In any process of change, no matter how tiny, before we seek to engage others in something new, it's important to honour the good intentions behind 'what we've always done' or 'what we're currently doing', and the people involved in upholding those systems. This is equally true when you meet as a 'tribe' to discuss tiny project first steps, and when you communicate out, formally (by email) or informally (chat on the ward) the tiny change you are exploring. This does two things: it lowers resistance from colleagues who might be naturally resistant to change, and from the system itself. William Bridges, veteran and acclaimed author on transition, talks about there being three key stages of transition, the first of which is endings or as he calls it 'when people identify what they are losing and learn how to manage these losses. They determine what is over and being left behind, and what they will keep. These may include relationships, processes, team members or locations.'[7] Reactions to the endings phase can include fear, denial, anger, sadness, disorientation, frustration, uncertainty, and a sense of loss.

So if my tiny project was enabling the midwife to be more 'with woman/family' in theatre and less 'with task', an endings phase might involve acknowledging and expressing gratitude for how our clearly defined roles in theatre have preserved safety for women and families; how any kind of change, no matter how small, disrupts the rhythm of what we know and may create fear or confusion; or a discussion over what is 'lost' when we share tasks more evenly, whether that's status, or control, or my (or his/her) established 'place' in the room. All this happens in the context of laying out a clear rationale for the tiny change.

This approach is very different from a top-down communication style: 'this change is happening for the good of the service, live with it'. It loses none of the clarity of purpose, but makes space for the people and feelings involved in transition.

If this sounds intimidating, remember you are not going it alone. You and your tribe are figuring this out, and you can take your time deciding how best to approach your tiny change.

### Start (with something) before you're ready

As a recovering perfectionist, the phrase 'start before you're ready' has been the most endorphin-boosting reminder to just try something, get something out there, start a conversation, refine and then try again.

> 'Do not wait until the conditions are perfect to begin. Beginning makes the conditions perfect. Do what you can, with what you have, where you are.' Attributed to Theodore Roosevelt

### Whatever you do, get started

> 'The secret of getting ahead is getting started. The secret of getting started is breaking your complex, overwhelming tasks into small manageable tasks, and then starting on the first one.' Attributed to Mark Twain

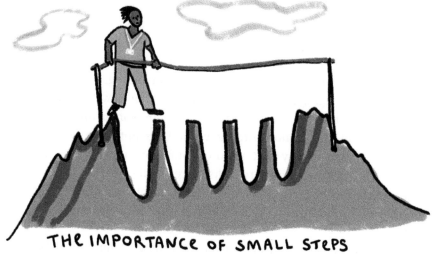

### THE IMPORTANCE OF SMALL STEPS

- Give yourselves permission – in your communication with others too – to try things out and not get it 'right', so that you can move closer to finding a way that works.
- Reframe feedback or feedforward (others' useful insights into how a situation can be improved in the future) as a gift. Ask for it. If it is constructive, we can build something with it, right!? Even if that's a new question to ask right now.

- Try not to be discouraged by the harder questions – they can generate possibility too. I find the phrasing in a John O'Donahue poem so helpful: 'the springtime edge of the bleak question.'[7]

## WHEN YOU FEEL OVERWHELMED

A reminder from *ikigai* for when we feel overwhelmed. *Ikigai,* the small, significant, often personal or humble pursuit of doing something you enjoy may offer the best of life.[9] Sometimes all we can do is focus on this.

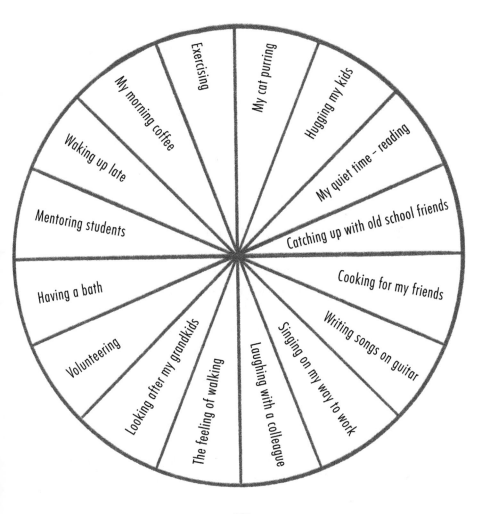

# CONCLUSION

# GOING FORWARD

## REALITY CHECK

This is not about doing it all ourselves and coming back into that cycle of self-flagellation and burnout.

It is actually about saying this: now I know more of who I am as a whole person and a midwife, who do I want to be, and what do I want to influence over the course of my career?

Now we have disentangled a little from the stories about ourselves, we may or may not echo the words of a midwife research participant 'A midwife is what I am. It's written through my body like a stick of rock.'[1] I love resilience researcher Lucie Warren's conviction that the greatest act of resilience might be to leave midwifery and choose another path.[2] These ways of being will help:

### Being kind, seeing and encouraging the whole person

> 'We must support and empower younger colleagues so that they will stay with us and not be frustrated by the realities of working in the NHS. ...I think the simplest things can empower them and make them feel good about themselves, this will surely help them to become more resilient...'[3]

### Being gentle with ourselves and aware of our relationship to the systems in which we work

> 'Part of the price for aiming high and "giving your all" while on duty is that occasionally you can't do the impossible. We must tell ourselves that it is the system that is failing, not us!'[4]

The reality is that when we are trying to change things, we often become more aware of what is broken. It can leave us feeling trapped between striving for tomorrow and losing hope in today, which can in turn lead to overwhelm and serve to detach us from our change work. So the quest becomes this: how might we hold our hopes for change lightly *and* stay connected to our purpose and to our allies, while recognising and embracing the jagged edges of our systems and services?

## Finding ongoing support

A critical friend might be part of this quest – someone who you can trust to be a thoughtful partner in this, or a small collective of peers all working on the same, or different, tiny change, big impact projects. What if you were to commit to rhythms of checking in – once a month for example – and revisiting your purpose (you could use the Big Why exercise on p.155 as a way of returning quickly to your purpose). There are examples throughout this book of people thinking differently about midwifery. Connect with them and others who care about the same things as you (see p.160 on connecting with your tribe). One of your ways of closing your monthly connection with a trusted partner or collective might be each of you naming three people to whom you are going to reach out that month, expanding your networks across midwifery and beyond. Strong bonds in your closer relationships are important – and weaker ties (via the networks you build) – are good too. The landscape of healthcare, social care and psychology practice, thinking and research is broad and exciting. You are invited.

## Keep having courageous conversations

Courageous conversations feel tough. They are the kind of conversations that feel risky but important. The conversation itself is a risk to the relationship but also vital to the relationship. A successful courageous conversation is one where, instead of putting on our armour, getting defensive or choosing to 'shut down' emotionally, we choose to stay open, curious and vulnerable. The other person may be encouraged to meet this with their own vulnerability where it's easier to get to the heart of the matter and say what needs to be said both ways. See the Resources Home for support on how to engage in courageous conversations, including an NHS Leadership Academy bitesize course.

## FINAL WORD

*'It is not the critic who counts: not the one who points out how the strong one stumbles or where the doer of deeds could have done better. The credit belongs to the one who is actually in the arena, whose face is marred by dust and sweat and blood, who strives valiantly, who errs and comes up short again and again... who spends herself for a worthy cause; who, at the best, knows, in the end, the triumph of high achievement, and who, at the worst, if she fails, at least she fails while daring greatly, so that her place shall never be with those cold and timid souls who knew neither victory nor defeat.'* Theodore Roosevelt 'Citizenship in a Republic' speech. Sorbonne, Paris, 23 April 1910

Teddy Roosevelt could have been speaking to us – so I've taken the liberty of rewording in the feminine, and adding my own emphasis to his famous words.

*You, brave soul and colleague, are*
*in the arena*
and
*daring greatly*
*already*
*by being here.*

The guidebook ends and the journey continues. If you have travelled with the guidebook alone so far, my hope is that you might find a trusted partner or small group to slowly go, and slowly grow, through the exercises in Part II and the reflective questions throughout Part I; that you might challenge each other to deeper depths and greater heights through trust and accountability.

You have experienced the breathless intensity of the journey through the oxygen-starved heights of the 'mega mountains' of our profession. Be gentle with yourself, especially if descriptions of trauma exposure, burnout or moral injury mirror your own experience. Use your discomfort as an opportunity to discuss the book with colleagues and leaders. Remember the respite and hope in Part I: text boxes asking 'What if…?', inviting us to take a deep breath from the oxygen canister and reimagine how we might take small, powerful steps to work and communicate differently. Use the 'What if…?' boxes, whoever you are, to open conversations with other midwives, support workers, your team, team leads, your director of midwifery. Find your tribe (p.159) and decide together what your small project for change might be.

And if that all feels too much, that's okay.

Revisiting the Part II exercises will not only resource you with a backpack full of strategies, tools, mindsets and resets, it will also bring a sense of clarity about who you are and your purpose as a midwife. This especially goes for the first section of Part II: passion and purpose. Investment in self-discovery here, with a partner, small group or coach, will serve you in every corner and every decade of your life.

Ultimately, my hope is that you stay in midwifery in a way that really works for you, or that you actively and joyously choose to leave. Either way will release you from the muddy waters of resentment between expectations (often unexamined and unexpressed) and disappointment.[5] Only when we collectively name what we really need does the system begin to shake.

Returning to Brené Brown's 'what if' question:

'What if, instead of looking at that person and saying what they are doing wrong or should be doing, I asked myself this question: What do I need but am afraid to ask for?'[6]

In a season of industrial action, this is a parallel call to action.

As Amanda Gorman described so movingly in her poem for the Biden inauguration, if we move forward rather than back, if we step into the light, unafraid and inspired, we will find hope and we will be able to value our differences and our scars.

*'For there is always light,
if only we're brave enough to see it'.*[7]

And be it.

The full poem is well worth reading and reflecting on after our journey together. [7]

I would love to hear how the book is helping you. Please connect @ wildrubiescoach and see flourishformidwives.com for additional resources. Make use of the carefully curated Resources Home too, at the end of the book.

## SOME FINAL REFLECTIVE QUESTIONS TO ENJOY

Finally, looking back over your learning from Part I and Part II, take some time to answer these questions:

- What territory have I taken? How far have I come?
- What valuable learning am I taking away?
- What commitments have I made?
- What will keep me on track?
- What is it to live life fully?
- What values require my attention to really live them?
- How will I now know to ask for support?
- How might I acknowledge myself right now?

## ABOUT THE AUTHOR

A midwife, coach and facilitator living in London, Kate seeks out green space, fresh air and wild water wherever she can. As a midwife she works within a continuity of carer team; as a coach she supports midwives and other bright sparks in healthcare to creatively reimagine their work lives. After a decade of pre-midwife life in Japan, Iran and the UAE, she loves that we all see the world from different angles. Her favourite part of being a midwife is witnessing and supporting 'newborn' families in their profound transition and changing identities. She brings an absolute conviction that there is no substitute in the world for you, and your unique voice.

Kate is a Certified Co-Active Coach (CPCC) and Professional Certified Coach (PCC) with the International Coach Federation (ICF). She is also a Firework licensed career coach and facilitator of Systemic Constellations. She's a skilled facilitator of groups, shaping leadership development environments for pioneering healthcare professionals, and enjoys creating reflective spaces with midwives and student midwives. She facilitates Schwartz Rounds (exploring the emotional impact of the work we do) for her home NHS trust. She holds an MA (Oxon) in Modern History, a DipHE in Antenatal Education and a BSc(Hons) in Midwifery.


## A NOTE ON DESCRIPTORS OF ETHNICITY

I have deliberately chosen, having taken the counsel of Black and Brown midwife colleagues, to use the descriptors Black, Brown and Mixed Ethnicity throughout the book, even when recounting statistics from an NHS report or survey which uses the terms BAME and BME. While the terms BAME or BME may be useful for defining a collective, they risk homogenising the stories, experiences and identities of distinctive groups. No label, even in the most nuanced research, is going to capture the realities, subtleties or unities of identity, but I recognise that the phrase ethnic minority or minorities risks further diminishing whole groups of people who have been intentionally minoritised by structural and institutional processes and systems. I have used the acronym BME only when it appears in the title of a report, for the sake of accurate citation.

# ACKNOWLEDGEMENTS

*'This is the high dream: that I might use all of who I am made
to be – the woman, the voice, the mother, the coach – to bring
refreshment and possibility to midwives who are losing hope. I am
not one to hold back, as you know, from thinking deep and wide,
believing anything is possible.'* 5 May 2017

I wrote this on International Day of the Midwife as I started my
midwifery journey in earnest. Thank you to the precious encouragers
and cheerleaders in my life, who have supported me through the
mountains and valleys of these years, and enabled this book to be
born. I guess I could call *all* of you midwives. Many of you are.

Thank you to my companion and sustainer God for the inspiration
to get on this path in the first place. You knew I'd come up with every
reason under the sun why it didn't make sense to go into midwifery,
so you found another way. Thank you for the timing of the 'little book'
picture you gave me on the last day of 2020. The emotional dark
days of the Covid peak January–March 2021 on the maternity wards,
hastened and sharpened the vision for finding a new way to name and
navigate the psychological impact of the work.

Andrew, you are the kindest and most gentle rock I know. Thank
you for sticking with me in sickness and in health. Hopefully you'll
be happy with the mountain analogy. Robin, Madeleine, Ione – I have
dedicated this book to you. Know that your births and early years reset
my life completely, and 'birthed' something in me beyond all I could
ask or imagine. Thank you. My dear sisters, mum and dad – thanks for
always believing in me. Mum – I'm sure you'll go on saying 'don't do
too much', and one day I might listen.

Thank you to my midwifery 'sistas' and 'mothers': Frances Barnsley,
my midwife for babies 1 and 3, thanks for being such a grounded
adventurer and staunch defender of all the best bits of true midwifery.
By the time this book is published it will be 20 years since I met you
with my naive eight-month bump. I trusted you completely. Sarah du
Feu, my godmother, midwife and artist, thank you for sowing an early
seed and watering it when it finally took root.

Sistas of the highest order: Effie Boorman, Maya Kemp, Sam

Perez-Amack, Katia Smith, Maeliss Preux, Josie Wood. Thank you for sharing life in such an intense way. When I think of you all, I think of some of the biggest raucous belly laughs I have ever had. Sistas beyond measure: Sophie Linghorn and Bryony Alcock. Without you (and Monty and Rosie) in Richmond Park, I couldn't have made sense of it all, or written this book. Sistas of vistas: Corrina Gordon-Barnes, Michaela Frances, Edith Graham and Cari Caldwell – we do perspective together. The view expands in coaching with you and I'll always be grateful. Sistas forever: Emma Croft, Angie Newby-Stubbs, Clare Benka, Michelle Campbell, Katie Madanat, Heather Coupland and Abi Sayers – thank you for your prayers and for holding up hope – always.

Thank you to everyone who has contributed to the content or style of the book in so many ways. I will name you in alphabetical order but know that your input via your wisdom or your words has been distinctive and powerful: Clare Benka, Sheena Byrom, Effie Boorman, Chris and Clem Cleave, Joanne Cull, Paula Cummins, Alice Dulson, Edith Graham, Mark Greenstock, Alex Heath, Kristina Hemon, Maya Kemp, Grace Mitchell, Sam Perez-Amack, Amity Reed, Rory Stewart, Dionne Taylor. One contributor has asked not to be named: you know who you are and how thankful we all are for your story.

Thank you for the many rich conversations on Zoom, in person or via email over the course of 18 months which have shaped the book. I am so grateful for the collective wisdom and research of this set of stars in the night sky, working for human flourishing in healthcare: Clare Cable, Clare Capito, Kevin Croft, Joanne Cull, Rita Dyson Harris, Edith Graham, Leah Hazard, Billie Hunter, Nikki Hill, Anna Kent, Kay King, Brendan McCormack, Jenny Patterson, Jess Read, Pauline Slade, Jan Smith, Helen Spiby, Lucie Warren, Cathy Warwick

Enormous thanks go to Jo Bradshaw for her exquisite illustrations and to Susan Last and Martin Wagner, my ever-patient team at Pinter & Martin.

# RESOURCES HOME

### Moral injury

Drs Wendy Dean and Simon Talbot, pioneers in the exploration of moral injury, with a portal to their podcast Moral Matters: www.fixmoralinjury.org

British Medical Association (BMA) article drawing on recent research on moral distress in the NHS www.bma.org.uk/advice-and-support/nhs-delivery-and-workforce/creating-a-healthy-workplace/moral-distress-in-the-nhs-and-other-organisations

Make Birth Better resource 'Am I Being Coercive?' to help us reflect on where we might be overstepping our own moral boundaries static1.squarespace.com/static/5ed8a1b746cc235b44a50be1/t/5f513d55247f1f797a16e3d4/1599159639127/Am+I+being+coercive.pdf

### Burnout

Are you showing signs of burnout? From the well-respected Headington Institute: www.headington-institute.org/resource/burnout-self-test/

Really drilling down to explore what is causing your burnout: www.headington-institute.org/resource/what-to-do-about-burnout-identifying-your-sources/

A guide to recognising and managing burnout from Thrive Worldwide: thrive-worldwide.org/wp-content/uploads/2022/06/Burnout.pdf

Helpful guide for all, including managers and leaders, about how to recognise signs of burnout and reduce symptoms and impact: proqol.org/burnout

Professional Quality of Life self-assessment for health workers measuring compassion satisfaction, compassion fatigue, and burnout – also offers resources designed to help: proqol.org/proqol-health-measure

Alessandra Pigni (2016) *The Idealist's Survival Kit: 75 Simple Ways to Avoid Burnout* Berkerley, CA: Parallax Press.

OnBeing podcast with Krista Tippett (2016): The Inner Life of Rebellion: how do we make activism sustainable? onbeing.org/programs/parker-palmer-courtney-martin-the-inner-life-of-rebellion/

### Compassion fatigue/empathic strain

Excellent TEDx talk The Edge of Compassion by Françoise Mathieu. Where is the sweet spot between caring too much and not caring at all? Also discusses our 'window of tolerance': www.youtube.com/watch?v=IcaUA6A37q8 (17:41)

Stirring TEDx talk Beyond the Cliff by Laura van Dernoot Lipsky about the impact of trauma exposure on our lives: www.youtube.com/watch?v=uOzDGrcvmus (19:23)

Resources from TEND Academy, working with high-stress and trauma-exposed individuals and workplaces: www.tendacademy.ca/resources

Compassion Fatigue Awareness Project and resources: www.compassionfatigue.org

A loving kindness meditation. 7 mins daily practice to reshape the brain: https://ggia.berkeley.edu/practice/loving_kindness_meditation

**Perinatal trauma-informed care**

Resources from the wonderful UK team at Make Birth Better www.makebirthbetter.org/what-is-birth-trauma and www.makebirthbetter.org/trauma-support-for-professionals. A video explanation of the Make Birth Better model is available at www.makebirthbetter.org/support-for-your-team and free downloads at www.makebirthbetter.org/free-downloads-professionals

A UK good practice guide to support implementation of trauma-informed care in the perinatal period with spotlight on the experience of women and families and recognition of the needs of staff: www.england.nhs.uk/wp-content/uploads/2021/02/BBS-TIC-V8.pdf

**Trauma exposure good practice**

Mental Health First Aid training for staff, building towards a peer-to-peer programme: mhfaengland.org/

If you are asking yourself the question 'where on earth would I start with helping to create an organisational or team culture of compassion?' use this helpful interactive pdf. from NHS England: www.england.nhs.uk/wp-content/uploads/2018/10/resource-pack-to-support-workplace-compassion-march-2020.pdf

Helping NHS leaders, teams and individuals to recover from the trauma of Covid-19 a compassionate approach from Avon and Wiltshire Mental Health Partnership NHS Trust: www.awp.nhs.uk/download_file/force/206/415

Really useful 2021 Scottish Trauma Informed Practice Toolkit exploring all aspects of a service https://www.gov.scot/publications/trauma-informed-practice-toolkit-scotland/

**Anti-racism starter resources**

Birthrights Report: Systemic Racism, not broken bodies: An inquiry into racial injustce and human rights in maternity care www.birthrights.org.uk/wp-content/uploads/2022/05/Birthrights-inquiry-systemic-racism-May-22-web-1.pdf

FiveXMore Report: The Black Maternity Experiences Survey: A Nationwide Study of Black Women's Experiences of Maternity Services in the United Kingdom: www.fivexmore.com

Capital Midwife Anti Racism Framework. Search under Health Education England (HEE) as it remains in xls. format for now.

David Williams is a social scientist at Harvard University. His TEDMED talk explores how racism impacts health: www.ted.com/talks/david_r_williams_how_racism_makes_us_sick (17:00)

Excellent list of anti-racism books, articles, podcasts, documentaries and more from Rise UK: www.riseuk.org.uk/resources/anti-racism-resources

Nova Reid's *The Good Ally*: www.novareid.com/the-good-ally/

Ibram X. Kendi's *How to be an Anti-Racist* and essays: www.ibramxkendi.com/essays

Reni Eddo-Lodge's *Why I'm no Longer Talking to White People About Race*: http://renieddolodge.co.uk and her About Race podcast: www.aboutracepodcast.com

TED talk: The Danger of a Single Story by Chimamanda Ngozi Adichie: www.ted.com/talks/chimamanda_ngozi_adichie_the_danger_of_a_single_story?referrer=playlist-how_to_tell_a_story (18:33)

White Privilege: Unpacking the Invisible Knapsack pdf by Peggy McIntosh: nationalseedproject.org/images/documents/Knapsack_plus_Notes-Peggy_McIntosh.pdf

Black Cultural Archives: Telling the story of the Black British Experience: artsandculture.google.com/project/black-cultural-archives

Richard Dyer's *White: Essays on Race and Culture*: www.routledge.com/White-Twentieth-Anniversary-Edition/Dyer/p/book/9781138683044

Peter Fryer's *Staying Power: The History of Black People in Britain*: www.plutobooks.com/9780745338309/staying-power/

Liberate Meditation app. Supporting the black community in developing a daily meditation practice.

**Sleep**

Matt Walker *Why We Sleep: The New Science of Sleep and Dreams* (2017) with some shocking insights into the impact of shift work and sleep deprivation. Access his podcast and TEDx talk Sleep is your Superpower at: www. sleepdiplomat.com/

Association of Anaesthetists Fight Fatigue Campaign and Resources, drawing on learning from other industries: https://anaesthetists.org/Home/Wellbeing-support/Fatigue/-Fight-Fatigue-download-our-information-packs

## Breathing

www.flourishformidwives.com for breathing exercises and visualisations

www.compassionatemind.co.uk/resource/audio. Some excellent audios of breathing exercises and visualisations

James Nestor's book *Breath: The New Science of a Lost Art* and talk 5 Ways to Improve Your Breathing: www.youtube.com/watch?v=f6yAY1oZUOA (11:57)

Headspace/Unmind apps for daily/shift go-to audios.

Professor Mark Williams' meditations/breathing space at: franticworld.com/resources/

## Being well

Self-compassion researcher Kristin Neff's site with a self-compassion test: self-compassion.org/self-compassion-test/ and exercises to develop self-compassion: self-compassion.org/category/exercises/#exercises

Simple and powerful Feet on the Floor grounding exercise from the TEND Academy: www.tendacademy.ca/feet-on-the-floor

Audios, videos and more from the Compassionate Mind Foundation, founded by Prof. Paul Gilbert and team as an international charity in 2006 www.compassionatemind.co.uk/resource/resources

Free access to the first 2 sessions of the One Thought online course with Aaron Turner, exploring the power of our mind in how we perceive and experience our environment at https://onethoughtonline.com

Sixty free tools from Karen Forshaw and Chrissie Mowbray's Resilience Toolkit at www.resilientpractice.co.uk/resilience-tools

Being Well podcast organised by topic so easy to search: www.rickhanson.net/being-well-podcast/being-well-podcast-by-topic/

Fascinating Facts about the Vagus Nerve and how to use it www.mentalfloss.com/article/65710/9-nervy-facts-about-vagus-nerve

CBT self-help and therapy resources: www.getselfhelp.co.uk

The Blurt Foundation: helping those affected by depression. Resources at www.blurtitout.org

All4Maternity online Nurture Zone. Subscription with online and print The Practising Midwife at https://www.all4maternity.com/caring/nurture/

### Being and knowing yourself

Free Via Institute Survey on your resources and internal strengths: www.viacharacter.org/

Free Myers Briggs based test and profiles: www.truity.com/test/type-finder-research-edition

An alternative Myers Briggs based personality instrument: www.16personalities.com/free-personality-test

DiSC based personality test and profiles: www.truity.com/test/disc-personality-test

Enneagram based style test and profiles: www.truity.com/test/enneagram-personality-test

A free saboteur awareness assessment - how we self-sabotage: www.positiveintelligence.com/saboteurs/

### Living and leading with compassion

Michael West on the core behaviours of compassionate leadership and the impact of experiencing ABC (Autonomy, Belonging and Control): www.youtube.com/watch?v=RrPmMwg9X8s (7:00)

How to have a wellbeing conversation from NHS Leadership Academy learninghub.leadershipacademy.nhs.uk/projectm_old_v1/wellbeing-conversations/

Business in the Community (BITC) has partnered with Public Health England to produce toolkits to help every organisation support the mental health and wellbeing of its employees. www.bitc.org.uk/ They also have a baseline wellbeing assessment tool.

The Compassion Institute offers an 8-week Compassion Cultivation Training programme, developed at Stanford University using evidenced based meditation techniques: www.compassioninstitute.com/ with links to audios to support Box Breathing and the Just Like Me exercise from Part II soundcloud.com/compassion-institute/sets/well-being-practices/s-SwFY4n8Nxno

The International Compassion Community curates an online space for those working in healthcare, with live daily guided meditations, webinars etc ccmm.care/meditations/

The King's Fund, a leading UK health and social care charity and think-tank offering blogs, videos, webinars on compassionate leadership www.kingsfund.org.uk/

Clinical psychologist Dr Deborah Lee leads a compassionate leadership course in the NHS which starts, of course, with self-awareness and self-compassion. Here she gives a talk entitled Everyone Needs Compassion vimeo.com/256389115 (17:00)

Emergency medicine Dr. Stephen Trzeciak's TEDx talk How 40 Seconds of Compassion Could Save a Life (including the life of the healthcare worker): www.youtube.com/watch?v=elW69hyPUuI (15:00)


**Working with challenge and vulnerability**

Adar Cohen, conflict resolution specialist TEDx talk, 3 ways to lead tough, unavoidable conversations: www.ted.com/talks/adar_cohen_3_ways_to_lead_tough_unavoidable_conversations?language=en (15:45)

Free NHS Leadership Academy bitesize course on courageous conversations: learninghub.leadershipacademy.nhs.uk/guides/courageous-conversations/

Brené Brown resources on tough conversations including the 'rumble' team process they use in her organisation: brenebrown.com/collections/a-courageous-approach-to-feedback/. Also see her book Dare to Lead: Brave Work. Tough Conversations. Whole Hearts (2018)

Amy Gallo's TEDx talk The Gift of Conflict with compassion and kindness: www.youtube.com/watch?v=MnaLS7OE2pk (14:47)

Harvard Business Review on Handling difficult conversations: hbr.org/2017/05/how-to-have-difficult-conversations-when-you-dont-like-conflict

US Society for Human Resource Management resources for dealing with 'difficult' people: www.shrm.org/hr-today/news/hr-magazine/0217/pages/how-do-you-deal-with-difficult-people.aspx

Otto Scharmer (MIT Presencing Institute, author of Theory U ottoscharmer.com ) on our four levels of listening: downloading, factual, empathic and generative listening: https://www.youtube.com/watch?v=eLfXpRkVZaI (8:25)

### Psychological safety

Developed in collaboration with Amy Edmondson of Harvard Business School. Describes the tool for measuring psychological safety: fearlessorganization. com

Building a psychologically safe workplace TEDx talk with Amy Edmondson: www.youtube.com/watch?v=LhoLuui9gX8 (11:25)

The difference between a 'real team' and a 'pseudo team' from Professor Michael West: www.youtube.com/watch?v=bqipJlb1oMM (2:16)

### Leadership at every level

NHS Leadership Academy's excellent inspiration library with videos and podcasts on cultural competence, courageous conversations, psychological safety and more: learninghub.leadershipacademy.nhs.uk/inspiration-library/

For scholarship, learning opportunities and community at the NHS Leadership Academy: www.leadershipacademy.nhs.uk/

Free mini courses on aspects of communication and leadership, including How to Run a 10 minute 'pause space': learninghub.leadershipacademy.nhs.uk/all-bitesize/

NHS kindness and positivity network: fabnhsstuff.net/fab-collections/kindness-positivity-campaign

Leadership resources from the Florence Nightingale Foundation: https://academy.florence-nightingale-foundation.org.uk. Also explore The Leadership Log podcast @leadership_log initiated by Florence Nightingale Foundation leadership programme scholars

Appreciative Inquiry short animation: www.youtube.com/watch?v=QzW22wwh1J4&t=71s (3:40). AI interview and reflective questions for your small change big impact project from the team at Positive Psychology positivepsychology.com/appreciative-inquiry-questions/

An animated introduction to systems thinking called In a World of Systems: www.youtube.com/watch?v=A_BtS008J0k&list=PLnVdw61jC-KBO-0LwEZSOP0ND48O6-jj4 (9:22)

Growing system leaders via the Academy for Change's Systems Fieldbook for Change: www.systemsfieldbook.org/foundational-ideas and a fantastic range of tools for self, team organisation and system at: www.systemsfieldbook.org/tools

# REFERENCES

**Love letter to Midwifery leaders**

1. Rizq R. The perversion of care: Psychological therapies in a time of IAPT. Psychodyn Pract [Internet]. 2012;18(1):7–24. Available from: http://dx.doi.org/10.1080/14753634.2012.640161

**Introduction**

1. Hunter B, Fenwick J, Sidebotham M, Henley J. Midwives in the United Kingdom: Levels of burnout, depression, anxiety and stress and associated predictors. *Midwifery* [Internet]. 2019;79(102526):102526. Available from: http://dx.doi.org/10.1016/j.midw.2019.08.008
2. Cull J, Hunter B, Henley J, Fenwick J, Sidebotham M. "Overwhelmed and out of my depth": Responses from early career midwives in the United Kingdom to the Work, Health and Emotional Lives of Midwives study. *Women Birth* [Internet]. 2020;33(6):e549–57. Available from: http://dx.doi.org/10.1016/j.wombi.2020.01.003
3. RCM. RCM warns of midwife exodus as maternity staffing crisis grows [Internet]. 2021. Available from: https://www.rcm.org.uk/media-releases/2021/september/rcm-warns-of-midwife-exodus-as-maternity-staffing-crisis-grows/
4. Cull J, Hunter B, Henley J, Fenwick J, Sidebotham M. "Overwhelmed and out of my depth": Responses from early career midwives in the United Kingdom to the Work, Health and Emotional Lives of Midwives study. *Women Birth* [Internet]. 2020;33(6):e549–57. Available from: http://dx.doi.org/10.1016/j.wombi.2020.01.003
5. Pezaro S, Maher K, Bailey E, Pearce G. Problematic substance use: an assessment of workplace implications in midwifery. *Occup Med* (Lond) [Internet]. 2021;71(9):460–6. Available from: http://dx.doi.org/10.1093/occmed/kqab127
6. Broughton E. Work stress made me self-harm: The grim state of UK midwifery [Internet]. Refinery29. 2022. Available from: https://www.refinery29.com/en-gb/2022/01/10808185/nhs-midwife-stress-burnout-uk
7. Ockenden D. Ockenden Report – Final Findings, Conclusions and Essential Actions from the Independent Review of Maternity Services at The Shrewsbury and Telford Hospital NHS Trust; March 2022. Available from: https://assets.publishing.service.gov.uk/government/uploads/system/uploads/attachment_data/file/1064302/Final-Ockenden-Report-web-accessible.pdf
8. West M, Dawson K, Kaur M. for The King's Fund. Making the Difference: Diversity and Inclusion in the NHS [Internet]. 2015. Available from: https://www.kingsfund.org.uk/sites/default/files/field/field_publication_file/Making-the-difference-summary-Kings-Fund-Dec-2015.pdf
9. Lord M. Being Black and birthing in the west. 2019 Sep; Available from: https://www.midwifery.org.uk/blog/bame-experience/being-black-and-birthing-in-the-west
10. RCM. BME midwives, disciplinary proceedings and the Workplace Race Equality Standard [Internet]. 2016. Available from: https://www.rcm.org.uk/media/5432/bme3.pdf
11. Reed A. *Overdue: Birth, burnout and a blueprint for a better NHS.* London, England: Pinter & Martin; 2020.
12. West M, Bailey S, Williams E. *The courage of compassion: Supporting nurses and midwives to deliver high-quality care.* London: The Kings Fund [Internet].

2020. Available from https://www.kingsfund.org.uk/sites/default/files/2020-09/The%20courage%20of%20compassion%20full%20report_0.pdf

13. Mestdagh E, Timmermans O, Fontein-Kuipers Y, Van Rompaey B. Proactive behaviour in midwifery practice: A qualitative overview based on midwives' perspectives. *Sex Reprod Healthc* [Internet]. 2019;20:87–92. Available from: http://dx.doi.org/10.1016/j.srhc.2019.04.002

14. Patterson E. *Reflect to create! The dance of reflection for creative leadership, professional practice and supervision: Reflective journal and workbook.* Centre for Reflection and Creativity Ltd; 2019

**Part I**

**Chapter 1: The current landscape: Hero or Villain: the problem of the status of midwife in the NHS and in popular culture**

1. UNFPA. Supporting Midwives: Our Frontline Heroes [Internet]. 2021. Available from: https://www.youtube.com/watch?v=yZgQPAL53K4

2. UNFPA. Supporting Midwives: Our Frontline Heroes [Internet]. 2021. Available from: https://www.youtube.com/watch?v=yZgQPAL53K4

3. Personal correspondence with newly qualified midwives, 2021

4. Osterholzer S. The Midwife's Husband, Part One [Internet]. 2018. Available from: https://www.kimosterholzer.com/22/midwifes-husband-part-one/

5. Kitzinger S. *Rediscovering Birth.* 2nd ed. London, England: Pinter & Martin; 2011.

6. Cambridge essential English dictionary 10th Edition: definition of vocation. Cambridge: Cambridge University Press; 2007.

7. Bloxsome D, Bayes S, Ireson D. "I love being a midwife; it's who I am": A Glaserian Grounded Theory Study of why midwives stay in midwifery. *J Clin Nurs* [Internet]. 2020;29(1–2):208–20. p213. Available from: http://dx.doi.org/10.1111/jocn.15078

8. Hunter B, Fenwick J, Sidebotham M, Henley J. Midwives in the United Kingdom: Levels of burnout, depression, anxiety and stress and associated predictors. *Midwifery* [Internet]. 2019;79(102526). Available from: http://dx.doi.org/10.1016/j.midw.2019.08.008

9. Batt-Rawden S. We need to stop calling NHS staff heroes – for a very important reason. *The Independent* [Internet]. 2021; Available from: https://www.independent.co.uk/voices/nhs-covid-stress-burnout-heroes-b1840683.html

10. Murray E, Kaufman KR, Williams R. Let us do better: learning lessons for recovery of healthcare professionals during and after COVID-19. *BJPsych Open* [Internet]. 2021;7(5):e151. Available from: http://dx.doi.org/10.1192/bjo.2021.981

11. Pezaro S, Clyne W, Turner A, Fulton EA, Gerada C. "Midwives Overboard!" Inside their hearts are breaking, their makeup may be flaking but their smile still stays on. *Women And Birth: Journal Of The Australian College Of Midwives.* 2016;29(3):e59–66. Available from: https://doi.org/10.1016/j.wombi.2015.10.006

12. Pezaro S, Clyne W, Fulton EA. A systematic mixed-methods review of interventions, outcomes and experiences for midwives and student midwives in work-related psychological distress. *Midwifery* [Internet]. 2017;50:163–73. Available from: http://dx.doi.org/10.1016/j.midw.2017.04.003

13. Smith J. *Nurturing Maternity Staff: How to tackle trauma, stress and burnout to create a positive working culture in the NHS.* London, England: Pinter & Martin; 2022.

14. Leversidge A. Why midwives leave – revisited. *Midwives.* 2016;19.

15. NHS Resolution: Annual Report and Accounts [Internet]. 2021-2022. Available

from: https://resolution.nhs.uk/wp-content/uploads/2022/07/NHS-Resolution-Annual-report-and-accounts-2021_22_Access.pdf

16. Cull J, Hunter B, Henley J, Fenwick J, Sidebotham M. "Overwhelmed and out of my depth": Responses from early career midwives in the United Kingdom to the Work, Health and Emotional Lives of Midwives study. *Women Birth* [Internet]. 2020;33(6):e549–57. MW323, pp.7. Available from: http://dx.doi.org/10.1016/j.wombi.2020.01.003

17. Mathieu F. *The compassion fatigue workbook: Creative tools for transforming compassion fatigue and vicarious traumatization.* New York: Routledge; 2012.

18. Morris R. How to Know if You're Being 'Resilience Victim Blamed'. You are not a Frog podcast Episode 145 with Dr Rachel Morris; 2022.

## Chapter 2: Occupational hazards

1. Pezaro S. "I suffer from a condition called being human." In: 3rd Annual Birth Trauma Conference 2018.

2. Coldridge L, Davies S. "Am I too emotional for this job?" An exploration of student midwives' experiences of coping with traumatic events in the labour ward. *Midwifery* [Internet]. 2017;45:1–6. Available from: http://dx.doi.org/10.1016/j.midw.2016.11.008

3. Coldridge L, Davies S. "Am I too emotional for this job?" An exploration of student midwives' experiences of coping with traumatic events in the labour ward. *Midwifery* [Internet]. 2017;45:1–6. Available from: http://dx.doi.org/10.1016/j.midw.2016.11.008

4. Warren L. personal communication; 2021

5. Hunter B, Warren L. Midwives' experiences of workplace resilience. *Midwifery* [Internet]. 2014;30(8):926–34. Available from: http://dx.doi.org/10.1016/j.midw.2014.03.010

6. NMC. Standards of Proficiency for Midwives [Internet]. 2019: p28. Available from: https://www.nmc.org.uk/globalassets/sitedocuments/standards/standards-of-proficiency-for-midwives.pdf

7. Ellis A. Changing rational-emotive therapy (RET) to rational emotive behavior therapy (REBT). *J Ration Emot Cogn Behav Ther* [Internet]. 1995;13(2):85–9. Available from: http://dx.doi.org/10.1007/bf02354453

8. NHS HEE: Reducing pre-registration attrition and improving retention [Internet]. Health Education England. 2018. Available from: https://www.hee.nhs.uk/our-work/reducing-pre-registration-attrition-improving-retention

9. Ockenden D. Ockenden Report – Final Findings, Conclusions and Essential Actions from the Independent Review of Maternity Services at The Shrewsbury and Telford Hospital NHS Trust; March 2022. Available from: https://assets.publishing.service.gov.uk/government/uploads/system/uploads/attachment_data/file/1064302/Final-Ockenden-Report-web-accessible.pdf

10. Hunter B, Warren L. Midwives' experiences of workplace resilience. *Midwifery* [Internet]. 2014;30(8):926–34. pp. 932-933. Available from: http://dx.doi.org/10.1016/j.midw.2014.03.010

## Chapter 3: Midwifery as emotion work

1. Hunter B, Deery R. Building our Knowledge about emotion work in midwifery, combining and comparing findings from two different research studies. *Evidence Based Midwifery* 2005; 3(1):10-15

2. Borrelli SE, Spiby H, Walsh D. The kaleidoscopic midwife: A conceptual metaphor illustrating first-time mothers' perspectives of a good midwife during childbirth. A grounded theory study. *Midwifery* [Internet]. 2016;39:103–

11. p103. Available from: http://dx.doi.org/10.1016/j.midw.2016.05.008

3.   Scamell M. The swan effect in midwifery talk and practice: a tension between normality and the language of risk: The swan effect in midwifery talk and practice. *Sociol Health Illn* [Internet]. 2011;33(7):987–1001. Available from: http://dx.doi.org/10.1111/j.1467-9566.2011.01366.x

4.   Reed R, Rowe J, Barnes M. Midwifery practice during birth: Ritual companionship. *Women Birth* [Internet]. 2016;29(3):269–78. Available from: http://dx.doi.org/10.1016/j.wombi.2015.12.003

5.   Newnham E, Kirkham M. Beyond autonomy: Care ethics for midwifery and the humanization of birth. *Nurs Ethics* [Internet]. 2019;26(7–8):2147–57. p.3. Available from: http://dx.doi.org/10.1177/0969733018819119

6.   Newnham E, Kirkham M. Beyond autonomy: Care ethics for midwifery and the humanization of birth. *Nurs Ethics* [Internet]. 2019;26(7–8):2147–57. p.3. Available from: http://dx.doi.org/10.1177/0969733018819119

7.   Hunter B. Conflicting ideologies as a source of emotion work in midwifery. *Midwifery* [Internet]. 2004;20(3):261–72. Available from: http://dx.doi.org/10.1016/j.midw.2003.12.004

8.   Cull J, Hunter B, Henley J, Fenwick J, Sidebotham M. "Overwhelmed and out of my depth": Responses from early career midwives in the United Kingdom to the Work, Health and Emotional Lives of Midwives study. *Women Birth* [Internet]. 2020;33(6):e549–57. MW 316 p4. Available from: http://dx.doi.org/10.1016/j.wombi.2020.01.003

9.   Scamell M. The swan effect in midwifery talk and practice: a tension between normality and the language of risk: The swan effect in midwifery talk and practice. *Sociol Health Illn* [Internet]. 2011;33(7):987–1001. p988. Available from: http://dx.doi.org/10.1111/j.1467-9566.2011.01366.x

10.  Scamell M. The swan effect in midwifery talk and practice: a tension between normality and the language of risk: The swan effect in midwifery talk and practice. *Sociol Health Illn* [Internet]. 2011;33(7):987–1001. p987. Available from: http://dx.doi.org/10.1111/j.1467-9566.2011.01366.x

11.  Cull J, Hunter B, Henley J, Fenwick J, Sidebotham M. "Overwhelmed and out of my depth": Responses from early career midwives in the United Kingdom to the Work, Health and Emotional Lives of Midwives study. *Women Birth* [Internet]. 2020;33(6):e549–57. MW 409: p5. Available from: http://dx.doi.org/10.1016/j.wombi.2020.01.003

12.  Pezaro S, Pearce G, Bailey E. Childbearing women's experiences of midwives' workplace distress: Patient and public involvement. *Br J Midwifery* [Internet]. 2018;26(10):659–69. Available from: http://dx.doi.org/10.12968/bjom.2018.26.10.659

## Chapter 4: Mega mountain 1: moral injury

1.   Čartolovni A, Stolt M, Scott PA, Suhonen R. Moral injury in healthcare professionals: A scoping review and discussion. *Nurs Ethics* [Internet]. 2021;28(5):590–602. Available from: http://dx.doi.org/10.1177/0969733020966776

2.   Dean W, Talbot S, Dean A. Reframing Clinician Distress: Moral Injury Not Burnout. Federal practitioner : for the health care professionals of the VA. DoD, and PHS. 2019;36(9):400–2. p.400. Available from: https://www.ncbi.nlm.nih.gov/pmc/articles/PMC6752815/

3.   Dean W, Talbot SG. Physicians aren't 'burning out.' They're suffering from moral injury [Internet]. STAT. 2019. Available from: https://www.statnews.com/2018/07/26/physicians-not-burning-out-they-are-suffering-moral-

injury/

4.   Murray E, Kaufman KR, Williams R. Let us do better: learning lessons for recovery of healthcare professionals during and after COVID-19. *BJPsych Open* [Internet]. 2021;7(5):e151. Available from: http://dx.doi.org/10.1192/bjo.2021.981

5.   Best J. Undermined and undervalued: how the pandemic exacerbated moral injury and burnout in the NHS. *BMJ* [Internet]. 2021;374:n1858. Available from: http://dx.doi.org/10.1136/bmj.n1858

6.   NSPCC. Statistics briefing: child sexual abuse Available at [Internet]. 2021 Mar. Available from: https://learning.nspcc.org.uk/media/1710/statistics-briefing-child-sexual-abuse.pdf

7.   Moncrieff G, Gyte GML, Dahlen HG, Thomson G, Singata-Madliki M, Clegg A, et al. Routine vaginal examinations compared to other methods for assessing progress of labour to improve outcomes for women and babies at term. *Cochrane Libr* [Internet]. 2022;2022(3). Available from: http://dx.doi.org/10.1002/14651858.cd010088.pub3

8.   Scamell M, Stewart M. Time, risk and midwife practice: the vaginal examination. *Health Risk Soc* [Internet]. 2014;16(1):84–100. Available from: http://dx.doi.org/10.1080/13698575.2013.874549

9.   Patterson J, Hollins Martin CJ, Karatzias T. Disempowered midwives and traumatised women: Exploring the parallel processes of care provider interaction that contribute to women developing Post Traumatic Stress Disorder (PTSD) post childbirth. *Midwifery* [Internet]. 2019;76:21–35. Available from: http://dx.doi.org/10.1016/j.midw.2019.05.010

10.  Shallow H. Untangling the Maternity Crisis. In: Edwards N, Mander R, Murphy-Lawless J, editors. Abingdon: Routledge; 2018. p. 66–74.

11.  Patterson J, Hollins Martin CJ, Karatzias T. Disempowered midwives and traumatised women: Exploring the parallel processes of care provider interaction that contribute to women developing Post Traumatic Stress Disorder (PTSD) post childbirth. *Midwifery* [Internet]. 2019;76:21–35. p. 28. Available from: http://dx.doi.org/10.1016/j.midw.2019.05.010

12.  Newnham E, Kirkham M. Beyond autonomy: Care ethics for midwifery and the humanization of birth. *Nurs Ethics* [Internet]. 2019;26(7–8):2147–57. Available from: http://dx.doi.org/10.1177/0969733018819119

13.  Katie, student midwife, personal communication 2022

14.  Morris D. Moral Injury in the UK Episode 24 Moral Matters podcast [Internet]. 2021. Available from: https://podcasts.apple.com/gb/podcast/moral-matters/id1529907905?i=1000532481534

15.  British Medical Association. Moral distress and moral injury: Recognising and tackling it for UK doctors. 2021 Jun; Available from: https://www.bma.org.uk/media/4209/bma-moral-distress-injury-survey-report-june-2021.pdf

16.  British Medical Association. Moral distress and moral injury: Recognising and tackling it for UK doctors. 2021 Jun; Available from: https://www.bma.org.uk/media/4209/bma-moral-distress-injury-survey-report-june-2021.pdf

17.  British Medical Association. Moral distress and moral injury: Recognising and tackling it for UK doctors. 2021 Jun; Available from: https://www.bma.org.uk/media/4209/bma-moral-distress-injury-survey-report-june-2021.pdf

18.  Murray E, Krahé C, Goodsman D. Are medical students in prehospital care at risk of moral injury? *Emerg Med J* [Internet]. 2018;35(10):590–4. Available from: http://dx.doi.org/10.1136/emermed-2017-207216

19.  Birthrights. Human Rights in Maternity Care [Internet]. 2019. Available from: https://birthrights.org.uk/wp-content/uploads/2019/03/Human-rights-in-

maternity-care-2019.pdf
20. Walker A. (2018) An apology. Used with permission. First published: https://www.all4maternity.com/the-system-and-the-struggle-a-midwives-apology/
21. Bartzak PJ. Moral Injury is the Wound: PTSD is the Manifestation. *Medsurg Nurs.* 2015;24(3):Suppl 10-1.
22. Murray H, Ehlers A. Cognitive therapy for moral injury in post-traumatic stress disorder. *Cogn Behav Therap* [Internet]. 2021;14(e8):e8. Available from: http://dx.doi.org/10.1017/S1754470X21000040
23. Williamson V, Murphy D, Phelps A, Forbes D, Greenberg N. Moral injury: the effect on mental health and implications for treatment. *Lancet Psychiatry* [Internet]. 2021;8(6):453–5. p.454. Available from: http://dx.doi.org/10.1016/S2215-0366(21)00113-9
24. Patterson J, Hollins Martin CJ, Karatzias T. Disempowered midwives and traumatised women: Exploring the parallel processes of care provider interaction that contribute to women developing Post Traumatic Stress Disorder (PTSD) post childbirth. *Midwifery* [Internet]. 2019;76:21–35. Available from: http://dx.doi.org/10.1016/j.midw.2019.05.010
25. Patterson J, Hollins Martin CJ, Karatzias T. Disempowered midwives and traumatised women: Exploring the parallel processes of care provider interaction that contribute to women developing Post Traumatic Stress Disorder (PTSD) post childbirth. *Midwifery* [Internet]. 2019;76:21–35. Available from: http://dx.doi.org/10.1016/j.midw.2019.05.010
26. Patterson J, Hollins Martin CJ, Karatzias T. Disempowered midwives and traumatised women: Exploring the parallel processes of care provider interaction that contribute to women developing Post Traumatic Stress Disorder (PTSD) post childbirth. *Midwifery* [Internet]. 2019;76:21–35. Available from: http://dx.doi.org/10.1016/j.midw.2019.05.010
27. Wilcock F. The Midwives' Cauldron Podcast: S3 Episode 1 [Internet]. 2021. Available from: https://podcasts.apple.com/gb/podcast/the-midwives-cauldron/id1523178579?i=1000538300015

**Chapter 5: Mega mountain 2: compassion fatigue**

1. Otzelberger A. Burning Out for People and Planet. Four dangerous self-care myths [Online] [Internet]. 2019. Available from: https://medium.com/the-good-jungle/burning-out-for-people-and-planet-four-dangerous-self-care-myths-85f2ad1357a
2. Otzelberger A. How to Confront Suffering (without shutting down your feelings) [Online] [Internet]. 2018. Available from: https://medium.com/the-good-jungle/how-to-confront-suffering-without-shutting-down-your-feelings-6f638c1bf31f
3. Schwartz Rounds description and training. Available from: https://www.pointofcarefoundation.org.uk/our-programmes/staff-experience/about-schwartz-rounds/
4. Rice H, Warland J. Bearing witness: midwives experiences of witnessing traumatic birth. *Midwifery* [Internet]. 2013;29(9):1056–63. Available from: http://dx.doi.org/10.1016/j.midw.2012.12.003
5. Sorenson C, Bolick B, Wright K, Hamilton R. Understanding compassion fatigue in healthcare providers: A review of current literature: Compassion fatigue in healthcare providers. *J Nurs Scholarsh* [Internet]. 2016;48(5):456–65. Available from: http://dx.doi.org/10.1111/jnu.12229
6. Baranowsky AB. The silencing response in clinical practice: On the road to dialogue. In: Figley CR, editor. *Treating compassion fatigue.* Abingdon: Brunner-

Routledge; 2002. p. 155–70.

7. Baranowsky AB. The silencing response in clinical practice: On the road to dialogue. In: Figley CR, editor. *Treating compassion fatigue*. Abingdon: Brunner-Routledge; 2002. p. 155–70.

8. Otzelberger A. How to Confront Suffering (without shutting down your feelings) [Online] [Internet]. 2018. Available from: https://medium.com/the-good-jungle/how-to-confront-suffering-without-shutting-down-your-feelings-6f638c1bf31f

9. Sorenson C, Bolick B, Wright K, Hamilton R. Understanding compassion fatigue in healthcare providers: A review of current literature: Compassion fatigue in healthcare providers. *J Nurs Scholarsh* [Internet]. 2016;48(5):456–65. Available from: http://dx.doi.org/10.1111/jnu.12229

10. Otzelberger A. Burning Out for People and Planet. Four dangerous self-care myths [Online] [Internet]. 2019. Available from: https://medium.com/the-good-jungle/burning-out-for-people-and-planet-four-dangerous-self-care-myths-85f2ad1357a

11. Singer T, Klimecki OM. Empathy and compassion. *Curr Biol* [Internet]. 2014;24(18):R875–8. Available from: http://dx.doi.org/10.1016/j.cub.2014.06.054

12. Heath A. personal communication; 2022

13. Heath A. personal communication; 2022

14. Heath A. personal communication; 2022

15. Heath A. personal communication; 2022

16. Goleman D, Davidson R. *Altered Traits: Science Reveals How Meditation Changes Your Mind, Brain, and Body*. New York, NY: Avery Publishing Group; 2018.

17. Rohan E, Bausch J. Climbing Everest: oncology work as an expedition in caring. *J Psychosoc Oncol* [Internet]. 2009;27(1):84–118. Available from: http://dx.doi.org/10.1080/07347330802616043

18. Mathieu F. *The compassion fatigue workbook: Creative tools for transforming compassion fatigue and vicarious traumatization*. New York: Routledge; 2012: p22.

## Chapter 6: Mega mountain 3: burnout

1. World Health Organization. International Statistical Classification of Diseases and Related Health Problems (11th ed; ICD-11). 24, QD85. 2019.

2. Freudenberger HJ. The staff burnout syndrome in alternative institutions. *Psychotherapy: Theory, Research, and Practice*. 1974;12:73–82.

3. Pines AM, Aronson E. *Career burnout: causes and cures*. New York: The Free Press; 1988.

4. World Health Organization. International Statistical Classification of Diseases and Related Health Problems. (11th ed; ICD-11). 24, QD85. 2019.

5. Hunter B. The importance of reciprocity in relationships between community-based midwives and mothers. *Midwifery*. 2006;22(4):308–22.

6. Creedy DK, Sidebotham M, Gamble J, Pallant J, Fenwick J. Prevalence of burnout, depression, anxiety and stress in Australian midwives: a cross-sectional survey. *BMC Pregnancy Childbirth* [Internet]. 2017;17(1):13. Available from: http://dx.doi.org/10.1186/s12884-016-1212-5

7. Patterson J, Hollins Martin CJ, Karatzias T. Disempowered midwives and traumatised women: Exploring the parallel processes of care provider interaction that contribute to women developing Post Traumatic Stress Disorder (PTSD) post childbirth. *Midwifery* [Internet]. 2019;76:21–35: p.26. Available from: http://dx.doi.org/10.1016/j.midw.2019.05.010

8.  Hunter B, Fenwick J, Sidebotham M, Henley J. Midwives in the United Kingdom: Levels of burnout, depression, anxiety and stress and associated predictors. *Midwifery* [Internet]. 2019;79:102526. Available from: http://dx.doi.org/10.1016/j.midw.2019.08.008

9.  NHS Staff Survey 2021 [Internet]. 2022. Available from: [online] https://www.nhsstaffsurveys.com/static/f5b196e5bf02b9e0c65f3820f586697d/ST21_National-briefing.pdf

10. NHS Staff Survey 2021 [Internet]. 2022. Available from: [online] https://www.nhsstaffsurveys.com/static/f5b196e5bf02b9e0c65f3820f586697d/ST21_National-briefing.pdf

11. NHS Staff Survey 2021 [Internet]. 2022. Available from: [online] https://www.nhsstaffsurveys.com/static/f5b196e5bf02b9e0c65f3820f586697d/ST21_National-briefing.pdf

12. RCM. RCM warms of midwife exodus as maternity staffing crisis grows [Internet]. 2021. Available from: https://www.rcm.org.uk/media-releases/2021/september/rcm-warns-of-midwife-exodus-as-maternity-staffing-crisis-grows/

13. Cull J, Hunter B, Henley J, Fenwick J, Sidebotham M. "Overwhelmed and out of my depth": Responses from early career midwives in the United Kingdom to the Work, Health and Emotional Lives of Midwives study. *Women Birth* [Internet]. 2020;33(6):e549–57: MW 503 p.4. Available from: http://dx.doi.org/10.1016/j.wombi.2020.01.003

14. Delgado C, Upton D, Ranse K, Furness T, Foster K. Nurses' resilience and the emotional labour of nursing work: An integrative review of empirical literature. *Int J Nurs Stud* [Internet]. 2017;70:71–88. Available from: http://dx.doi.org/10.1016/j.ijnurstu.2017.02.008

15. Kinman G, Leggetter S. Emotional labour and wellbeing: What protects nurses? *Healthcare* 2016;4(4):89. https://www.ncbi.nlm.nih.gov/pmc/articles/PMC5198131/

16. Kinman G, Teoh K, Harriss A. *The Mental Health and Wellbeing of Nurses and Midwives in the United Kingdom.* London: The Society of Occupational Medicine. 2020. Available from: https://www.som.org.uk/sites/som.org.uk/files/The_Mental_Health_and_Wellbeing_of_Nurses_and_Midwives_in_the_United_Kingdom.pdf

17. Hunter B, Fenwick J, Sidebotham M, Henley J. Midwives in the United Kingdom: Levels of burnout, depression, anxiety and stress and associated predictors. *Midwifery* [Internet]. 2019;79(102526):102526. Available from: http://dx.doi.org/10.1016/j.midw.2019.08.008

18. Pezaro S, Maher K, Bailey E, Pearce G. Problematic substance use: an assessment of workplace implications in midwifery. *Occup Med* (Lond) [Internet]. 2021;71(9):460–6. Available from: http://dx.doi.org/10.1093/occmed/kqab127

19. Ross, CA, Berry, NS, Smye, V, Goldner, EM. A critical review of knowledge on nurses with problematic substance use: The need to move from individual blame to awareness of structural factors. *Nurs Inq.* 2018; 25:e12215. Available from: https://doi.org/10.1111/nin.12215

20. Vayr F, Herin F, Jullian B, Soulat JM, Franchitto N. Barriers to seeking help for physicians with substance use disorder: a review. *Drug and Alcohol Dependence* 2019;*199*:116–121. Available from: https://doi.org/10.1016/j.drugalcdep.2019.04.004

21. Hichisson AD, Corkery JM. Alcohol/substance use and occupational/post-traumatic stress in paramedics. *J Paramedic Pr* [Internet]. 2020;12(10):388–96.

Available from: http://dx.doi.org/10.12968/jpar.2020.12.10.388

22. Pezaro S, Maher K, Bailey E, Pearce G. Problematic substance use: an assessment of workplace implications in midwifery. *Occup Med* (Lond) [Internet]. 2021;71(9):460–6. Available from: http://dx.doi.org/10.1093/occmed/kqab127

23. Reed A. personal communication; 2021

24. van Dernoot Lipsky L, Burk C. *Trauma stewardship: An everyday guide to caring for self while caring for others.* San Francisco, CA: Berrett-Koehler; 2009: p81

25. Cull J, Hunter B, Henley J, Fenwick J, Sidebotham M. "Overwhelmed and out of my depth": Responses from early career midwives in the United Kingdom to the Work, Health and Emotional Lives of Midwives study. *Women Birth* [Internet]. 2020;33(6):e549–57: MW 452 pp.6. Available from: http://dx.doi.org/10.1016/j.wombi.2020.01.003

26. Cull J, Hunter B, Henley J, Fenwick J, Sidebotham M. "Overwhelmed and out of my depth": Responses from early career midwives in the United Kingdom to the Work, Health and Emotional Lives of Midwives study. *Women Birth* [Internet]. 2020;33(6):e549–57: MW 135 pp.4 Available from: http://dx.doi.org/10.1016/j.wombi.2020.01.003

27. Tresidder A. Denial, displacement and other ways we neglect ourselves with Dr Andrew Tresidder. You are not a Frog podcast Episode 77 with Dr Rachel Morris; 2019.

28. Yoshida Y, Sandall J. Occupational burnout and work factors in community and hospital midwives: a survey analysis. *Midwifery* [Internet]. 2013;29(8):921–6. Available from: http://dx.doi.org/10.1016/j.midw.2012.11.002

29. Sorby A. RCM: Midwives skipping breaks and working overtime [Internet]. 2020. Available at: https://www.rcm.org.uk/news-views/rcm-opinion/2020/midwives-skipping-breaks-and-working-overtime/

30. Cull J. personal communication; 2021

31. D'Annibale M, Hornzee N, Whelan M, Guess N, Hall W, Gibson R. Eating on the night shift: A need for evidence‐based dietary guidelines? *Nutr Bull* [Internet]. 2021;46(3):339–49. Available from: http://dx.doi.org/10.1111/nbu.12515

32. Reynolds AC, Paterson JL, Ferguson SA, Stanley D, Wright KP Jr, Dawson D. The shift work and health research agenda: Considering changes in gut microbiota as a pathway linking shift work, sleep loss and circadian misalignment, and metabolic disease. *Sleep Med Rev* [Internet]. 2017;34:3–9. Available from: http://dx.doi.org/10.1016/j.smrv.2016.06.009

33. Liu W, Zhou Z, Dong D, Sun L, Zhang G. Sex differences in the association between night shift work and the risk of cancers: A meta-analysis of 57 articles. *Dis Markers* [Internet]. 2018;2018:1–20. Available from: http://dx.doi.org/10.1155/2018/7925219

34. Gao Y, Gan T, Jiang L, Yu L, Tang D, Wang Y, et al. Association between shift work and risk of type 2 diabetes mellitus: a systematic review and dose-response meta-analysis of observational studies. *Chronobiol Int* [Internet]. 2020;37(1):29–46. Available from: http://dx.doi.org/10.1080/07420528.2019.1683570

35. Wang Y, Yu L, Gao Y, Jiang L, Yuan L, Wang P, et al. Association between shift work or long working hours with metabolic syndrome: a systematic review and dose-response meta-analysis of observational studies. *Chronobiol Int* [Internet]. 2021;38(3):318–33. Available from: http://dx.doi.org/10.1080/07420528.2020.1797763

36. Manohar S, Thongprayoon C, Cheungpasitporn W, Mao MA, Herrmann SM. Associations of rotational shift work and night shift status with hypertension: a

systematic review and meta-analysis. *J Hypertens* [Internet]. 2017;35(10):1929–37. Available from: http://dx.doi.org/10.1097/HJH.0000000000001442

37.  Boivin DB, Boudreau P, Kosmadopoulos A. Disturbance of the circadian system in shift work and its health impact. *J Biol Rhythms* [Internet]. 2022;37(1):3–28. Available from: http://dx.doi.org/10.1177/07487304211064218

38.  Fernandez Renae C, Vivienne M, Marino Jennifer M, Whitrow Melissa L, Michael D. Night Shift Among Women: Is It Associated With Difficulty Conceiving a First Birth? *Frontiers in Public Health* [Internet]. 2020;8. Available from: https://www.frontiersin.org/article/10.3389/fpubh.2020.595943

39.  Angerer P, Schmook R, Elfantel I, Li J. Night work and the risk of depression. *Dtsch Arztebl Int* [Internet]. 2017; Available from: http://dx.doi.org/10.3238/arztebl.2017.0404

40.  Torquati L, Mielke GI, Brown WJ, Burton NW, Kolbe-Alexander TL. Shift work and poor mental health: A meta-analysis of longitudinal studies. *Am J Public Health* [Internet]. 2019;109(11):e13–20. Available from: http://dx.doi.org/10.2105/ajph.2019.305278

41.  Reed A. personal communication; 2021

42.  Mollart L, Skinner VM, Newing C, Foureur M. Factors that may influence midwives work-related stress and burnout. *Women Birth* [Internet]. 2013;26(1):26–32. Available from: http://dx.doi.org/10.1016/j.wombi.2011.08.002

43.  West MA. *Effective Teamwork: Practical lessons from organisational research.* 3rd edition. Oxford: Blackwell Publishing; 2012

44.  Hunter B, Fenwick J, Sidebotham M, Henley J. Midwives in the United Kingdom: Levels of burnout, depression, anxiety and stress and associated predictors. *Midwifery* [Internet]. 2019;79(102526):102526. Available from: http://dx.doi.org/10.1016/j.midw.2019.08.008

45.  Cull J, Hunter B, Henley J, Fenwick J, Sidebotham M. "Overwhelmed and out of my depth": Responses from early career midwives in the United Kingdom to the Work, Health and Emotional Lives of Midwives study. *Women Birth* [Internet]. 2020;33(6):e549–57. Available from: http://dx.doi.org/10.1016/j.wombi.2020.01.003

46.  NHS England. NHS Staff Survey Results 2021: detailed spreadsheets. Available from: https://www.nhsstaffsurveys.com/results/national-results/

47.  Lyubovnikova J, West MA, Dawson JF, Carter MR. 24-karat or fool's gold? Consequences of real team and co-acting group membership in healthcare Organisations. *European Journal of Work and Organisational Psychology* 2015: 24 (6), 929-950. Available from: https://doi.org/10.1080/1359432X.2014.992421

48.  NHS England. NHS Staff Survey Results 2021: detailed spreadsheets. Available from: https://www.nhsstaffsurveys.com/results/national-results/

49.  West MA. *Compassionate Leadership: Sustaining Wisdom, Humanity and Presence in Health and Social Care.* London: The Swirling Leaf Press; 2021

50.  Lyubovnikova J, West MA, Dawson JF, Carter MR. 24-karat or fool's gold? Consequences of real team and co-acting group membership in healthcare Organisations. *European Journal of Work and Organisational Psychology* 2015: 24 (6), 929-950. Available from: https://doi.org/10.1080/1359432X.2014.992421

51.  Midwife, Anonymous. All4Maternity [Internet] 2018. Available from https://www.all4maternity.com/i-am-a-midwife-and-i-am-broken/

52.  Kitson-Reynolds E. *The Lived Experience of Newly Qualified Midwives.* [School of Health Sciences]: University of Southampton; 2010.

53.  Amir Z, Reid AJ. Impact of traumatic perinatal events on burnout rates among midwives. *Occup Med* (Lond) [Internet]. 2020;70(8):602–5. Available from: http://dx.doi.org/10.1093/occmed/kqaa156

54. Hazard L. Emma Gannon Ctrl Alt Delete podcast #213 Leah Hazard: Burnout in the NHS. 22 Aug 2019.

55. Sheen K, Slade P, Spiby H. An integrative review of the impact of indirect trauma exposure in health professionals and potential issues of salience for midwives. *J Adv Nurs* [Internet]. 2014;70(4):729–43. Available from: http://dx.doi.org/10.1111/jan.12274

56. Hunter B, Fenwick J, Sidebotham M, Henley J. Midwives in the United Kingdom: Levels of burnout, depression, anxiety and stress and associated predictors. *Midwifery* [Internet]. 2019;79(102526):102526. Available from: http://dx.doi.org/10.1016/j.midw.2019.08.008

57. Hildingsson I, Fenwick J. Swedish midwives' perception of their practice environment - A cross sectional study. *Sex Reprod Healthc* [Internet]. 2015;6(3):174–81. Available from: http://dx.doi.org/10.1016/j.srhc.2015.02.001

58. Hunter B. Conflicting ideologies as a source of emotion work in midwifery. *Midwifery* [Internet]. 2004;20(3):261–72. Available from: http://dx.doi.org/10.1016/j.midw.2003.12.004

59. Cull J, Hunter B, Henley J, Fenwick J, Sidebotham M. "Overwhelmed and out of my depth": Responses from early career midwives in the United Kingdom to the Work, Health and Emotional Lives of Midwives study. *Women Birth* [Internet]. 2020;33(6):e549–57. Available from: http://dx.doi.org/10.1016/j.wombi.2020.01.003

60. Hunter B, Warren L. Midwives' experiences of workplace resilience. *Midwifery* [Internet]. 2014;30(8):926–34. Available from: http://dx.doi.org/10.1016/j.midw.2014.03.010

61. Yoshida Y, Sandall J. Occupational burnout and work factors in community and hospital midwives: a survey analysis. *Midwifery* [Internet]. 2013;29(8):921–6. Available from: http://dx.doi.org/10.1016/j.midw.2012.11.002

62. Hunter B, Fenwick J, Sidebotham M, Henley J. Midwives in the United Kingdom: Levels of burnout, depression, anxiety and stress and associated predictors. *Midwifery* [Internet]. 2019;79(102526):102526. Available from: http://dx.doi.org/10.1016/j.midw.2019.08.008

63. Evans J, Taylor J, Browne J, Ferguson S, Atchan M, Maher P, et al. The future in their hands: Graduating student midwives' plans, job satisfaction and the desire to work in midwifery continuity of care. *Women Birth* [Internet]. 2020;33(1):e59–66. Available from: http://dx.doi.org/10.1016/j.wombi.2018.11.011

64. Yoshida Y, Sandall J. Occupational burnout and work factors in community and hospital midwives: a survey analysis. *Midwifery* [Internet]. 2013;29(8):921–6. Available from: http://dx.doi.org/10.1016/j.midw.2012.11.002

65. Cull J, Hunter B, Henley J, Fenwick J, Sidebotham M. "Overwhelmed and out of my depth": Responses from early career midwives in the United Kingdom to the Work, Health and Emotional Lives of Midwives study. *Women Birth* [Internet]. 2020;33(6):e549–57. Available from: http://dx.doi.org/10.1016/j.wombi.2020.01.003

66. Mollart L, Skinner VM, Newing C, Foureur M. Factors that may influence midwives work-related stress and burnout. *Women Birth* [Internet]. 2013;26(1):26–32. Available from: http://dx.doi.org/10.1016/j.wombi.2011.08.002

67. Bloxsome D, Bayes S, Ireson D. "I love being a midwife; it's who I am": A Glaserian Grounded Theory Study of why midwives stay in midwifery. *J Clin Nurs* [Internet]. 2020;29(1–2):208–20. Available from: http://dx.doi.org/10.1111/jocn.15078

68. Cull J, Hunter B, Henley J, Fenwick J, Sidebotham M. "Overwhelmed and out

of my depth": Responses from early career midwives in the United Kingdom to the Work, Health and Emotional Lives of Midwives study. *Women Birth* [Internet]. 2020;33(6):e549–57. Available from: http://dx.doi.org/10.1016/j.wombi.2020.01.003

69. Mestdagh E, Timmermans O, Fontein-Kuipers Y, Van Rompaey B. Proactive behaviour in midwifery practice: A qualitative overview based on midwives' perspectives. *Sex Reprod Healthc* [Internet]. 2019;20:87–92. Available from: http://dx.doi.org/10.1016/j.srhc.2019.04.002

70. Hunter B, Warren L. Midwives' experiences of workplace resilience. *Midwifery* [Internet]. 2014;30(8):926–34. Available from: http://dx.doi.org/10.1016/j.midw.2014.03.010

71. Kinman G, Teoh K, Harriss A. *The Mental Health and Wellbeing of Nurses and Midwives in the United Kingdom*. London: The Society of Occupational Medicine. 2020. Available from: https://www.som.org.uk/sites/som.org.uk/files/The_Mental_Health_and_Wellbeing_of_Nurses_and_Midwives_in_the_United_Kingdom.pdf

72. Slade P, Sheen K, Collinge S, Butters J, Spiby H. A programme for the prevention of post-traumatic stress disorder in midwifery (POPPY): indications of effectiveness from a feasibility study. *Eur J Psychotraumatol* [Internet]. 2018;9(1):1518069. Available from: http://dx.doi.org/10.1080/20008198.2018.1518069

**Chapter 7: Mega mountain 4: trauma exposure**

1. Rice H, Warland J. Bearing witness: midwives experiences of witnessing traumatic birth. *Midwifery* [Internet]. 2013;29(9):1056–63. Available from: http://dx.doi.org/10.1016/j.midw.2012.12.003

2. Sheen K, Spiby H, Slade P. Exposure to traumatic perinatal experiences and posttraumatic stress symptoms in midwives: prevalence and association with burnout. *Int J Nurs Stud* [Internet]. 2015;52(2):578–87. Available from: http://dx.doi.org/10.1016/j.ijnurstu.2014.11.006

3. Porges SW. The polyvagal theory: new insights into adaptive reactions of the autonomic nervous system. *Cleve Clin J Med* [Internet]. 2009;76 Suppl 2(4 suppl 2):S86-90. Available from: http://dx.doi.org/10.3949/ccjm.76.s2.17

4. Garratt L. *Survivors of Childhood Sexual Abuse and Midwifery Practice: CSA, Birth and Powerlessness*. London, England: Routledge; 2011.

5. Garratt L. *Survivors of Childhood Sexual Abuse and Midwifery Practice: CSA, Birth and Powerlessness*. London, England: Routledge; 2011: p.136

6. Garratt L. *Survivors of Childhood Sexual Abuse and Midwifery Practice: CSA, Birth and Powerlessness*. London, England: Routledge; 2011.

7. Garratt L. *Survivors of Childhood Sexual Abuse and Midwifery Practice: CSA, Birth and Powerlessness*. London, England: Routledge; 2011: p.136

8. Garratt L. *Survivors of Childhood Sexual Abuse and Midwifery Practice: CSA, Birth and Powerlessness*. London, England: Routledge; 2011.

9. Van Der Kolk B. *The Body Keeps the Score: Mind Brain and Body in the Transformation of Trauma*. London: Penguin; 2015.

10. Keane F. *Living with PTSD*. BBC Two documentary. Thu 26 May 2022.

11. Nott D. *War Doctor: Surgery on the front line*. London, London: Picador; 2020.

12. Kent A. *Frontline midwife: My story of survival and keeping others safe*. London, England: Bloomsbury Publishing Plc; 2022.

13. Pezaro S, Clyne W, Turner A, Fulton EA, Gerada C. "Midwives Overboard!" Inside their hearts are breaking, their makeup may be flaking but their smile still stays on. *Women And Birth: Journal of The Australian College of Midwives*.

2016;29(3):e59–66.

14. Leinweber J, Creedy DK, Rowe H, Gamble J. Responses to birth trauma and prevalence of posttraumatic stress among Australian midwives. *Women Birth* [Internet]. 2017;30(1):40–5. Available from: http://dx.doi.org/10.1016/j.wombi.2016.06.006

15. Cohen R, Leykin D, Golan-Hadari D, Lahad M. Exposure to traumatic events at work, posttraumatic symptoms and professional quality of life among midwives. *Midwifery* [Internet]. 2017;50:1–8. Available from: http://dx.doi.org/10.1016/j.midw.2017.03.009

16. Toohill J, Fenwick J, Sidebotham M, Gamble J, Creedy DK. Trauma and fear in Australian midwives. *Women Birth* [Internet]. 2019;32(1):64–71. Available from: http://dx.doi.org/10.1016/j.wombi.2018.04.003

17. Sheen K, Spiby H, Slade P. What are the characteristics of perinatal events perceived to be traumatic by midwives? *Midwifery* [Internet]. 2016;40:55–61. Available from: http://dx.doi.org/10.1016/j.midw.2016.06.007

18. Sheen K, Spiby H, Slade P. What are the characteristics of perinatal events perceived to be traumatic by midwives? *Midwifery* [Internet]. 2016;40:55–61. Available from: http://dx.doi.org/10.1016/j.midw.2016.06.007

19. Patterson J, Hollins Martin CJ, Karatzias T. Disempowered midwives and traumatised women: Exploring the parallel processes of care provider interaction that contribute to women developing Post Traumatic Stress Disorder (PTSD) post childbirth. *Midwifery* [Internet]. 2019;76:21–35. Available from: http://dx.doi.org/10.1016/j.midw.2019.05.010

20. Beck CT, LoGiudice J, Gable RK. A mixed-methods study of secondary traumatic stress in certified nurse-midwives: Shaken belief in the birth process. *J Midwifery Womens Health* [Internet]. 2015;60(1):16–23. Available from: http://dx.doi.org/10.1111/jmwh.12221

21. Leinweber J, Creedy DK, Rowe H, Gamble J. A socioecological model of posttraumatic stress among Australian midwives. *Midwifery* [Internet]. 2017;45:7–13. Available from: http://dx.doi.org/10.1016/j.midw.2016.12.001

22. Sheen K, Spiby H, Slade P. Exposure to traumatic perinatal experiences and posttraumatic stress symptoms in midwives: prevalence and association with burnout. *Int J Nurs Stud* [Internet]. 2015;52(2):578–87. Available from: http://dx.doi.org/10.1016/j.ijnurstu.2014.11.006

23. Wahlberg Å, Andreen Sachs M, Johannesson K, Hallberg G, Jonsson M, Skoog Svanberg A, et al. Post-traumatic stress symptoms in Swedish obstetricians and midwives after severe obstetric events: a cross-sectional retrospective survey. *BJOG* [Internet]. 2017;124(8):1264–71. Available from: http://dx.doi.org/10.1111/1471-0528.14259

24. Mathieu F. *The compassion fatigue workbook: Creative tools for transforming compassion fatigue and vicarious traumatization.* New York: Routledge; 2012.

25. Bullock, M. Public Health Speciality Registrar Greater London Authority. Adverse Childhood Experiences in London: Investigating ways that Adverse Childhood Experiences and related concepts of vulnerability can help us to understand and improve Londoners' health [Internet]. 2019. Available from: https://www.london.gov.uk/sites/default/files/adverse_childhood_experiences_in_london._final_report_october_2019_with_author._mb.pdf

26. NSPCC. Statistics briefing: child sexual abuse Available at [Internet]. 2021 Mar. Available from: https://learning.nspcc.org.uk/media/1710/statistics-briefing-child-sexual-abuse.pdf [Accessed 09/09/2021]

27. Office for National Statistics. Crime Survey for England and Wales: domestic abuse prevalence dataset [Internet]. 2020. Available from: https://www.

ons.gov.uk/peoplepopulationandcommunity/crimeandjustice/datasets/
domesticabuseprevalenceandvictimcharacteristicsappendixtables

28. Beck CT, LoGiudice J, Gable RK. A mixed-methods study of secondary traumatic stress in certified nurse-midwives: Shaken belief in the birth process. *J Midwifery Womens Health* [Internet]. 2015;60(1):16–23. Available from: http://dx.doi.org/10.1111/jmwh.12221

29. Leinweber J, Creedy DK, Rowe H, Gamble J. Responses to birth trauma and prevalence of posttraumatic stress among Australian midwives. *Women Birth* [Internet]. 2017;30(1):40–5. Available from: http://dx.doi.org/10.1016/j.wombi.2016.06.006

30. Kay A. *This is Going to Hurt*. BBC productions; 2022.

31. van Dernoot Lipsky L, Burk C. *Trauma stewardship: An everyday guide to caring for self while caring for others*. San Francisco, CA: Berrett-Koehler; 2009: pp 43-44

32. Dahlen HG, Caplice S. What do midwives fear? *Women Birth* [Internet]. 2014;27(4):266–70. Available from: http://dx.doi.org/10.1016/j.wombi.2014.06.008

33. Christoffersen L, Teigen J, Rønningstad C. Following-up midwives after adverse incidents: How front-line management practices help second victims. *Midwifery* [Internet]. 2020;85:102669: Participant 17 p.5. Available from: http://dx.doi.org/10.1016/j.midw.2020.102669

34. Minooee S, Cummins A, Foureur M, Travaglia J. Catastrophic thinking: Is it the legacy of traumatic births? Midwives' experiences of shoulder dystocia complicated births. *Women Birth* [Internet]. 2021;34(1):e38–46. Available from: http://dx.doi.org/10.1016/j.wombi.2020.08.008

35. Christoffersen L, Teigen J, Rønningstad C. Following-up midwives after adverse incidents: How front-line management practices help second victims. *Midwifery* [Internet]. 2020;85(102669):102669. Available from: http://dx.doi.org/10.1016/j.midw.2020.102669

36. Leinweber J, Rowe HJ. The costs of "being with the woman": secondary traumatic stress in midwifery. *Midwifery* [Internet]. 2010;26(1):76–87. Available from: http://dx.doi.org/10.1016/j.midw.2008.04.003

37. Figley CR. Compassion fatigue as secondary traumatic stress disorder: an overview. Chapter 1of *Compassion Fatigue: coping with secondary traumatic stress disorder in those who treat the traumatized*. Figley CR, editor. New York: Brunner-Routledge; 1995: p.10.

38. Mathieu F. *The compassion fatigue workbook: Creative tools for transforming compassion fatigue and vicarious traumatization*. New York: Routledge; 2012: p14.

39. Mollart L, Newing C, Foureur M. Midwives' emotional wellbeing: Impact of conducting a Structured Antenatal Psychosocial Assessment (SAPSA). *Women Birth* [Internet]. 2009;22(3):82–8. Available from: http://dx.doi.org/10.1016/j.wombi.2009.02.001

40. Mathieu F. *The compassion fatigue workbook: Creative tools for transforming compassion fatigue and vicarious traumatization*. New York: Routledge; 2012.

41. Leap N, Hunter B. *The midwife's tale: An oral history from handywoman to professional midwife*. Barnsley, England: Pen & Sword Books; 2013.

42. Mathieu F. *The compassion fatigue workbook: Creative tools for transforming compassion fatigue and vicarious traumatization*. New York: Routledge; 2012.

43. Cohen R, Leykin D, Golan-Hadari D, Lahad M. Exposure to traumatic events at work, posttraumatic symptoms and professional quality of life among midwives. *Midwifery* [Internet]. 2017;50:1–8. Available from: http://dx.doi.

org/10.1016/j.midw.2017.03.009

44. Thomas R, Wilson J. Issues and controversies in the understanding and diagnosis of compassion fatigue, vicarious traumatisation and secondary traumatic stress disorder. *International Journal of Emergency Mental Health.* 2004;6:81–92.

45. Leinweber J, Rowe HJ. The costs of "being with the woman": secondary traumatic stress in midwifery. *Midwifery* [Internet]. 2010;26(1):76–87. Available from: http://dx.doi.org/10.1016/j.midw.2008.04.003

46. Midwife, one-year post-qualification. Personal communication; 2021.

47. Newly-qualified midwife. Personal communication; 2021.

**Chapter 8: Mega mountain 5: post-traumatic stress injury and the brain**

1. Sheen K, Spiby H, Slade P. Exposure to traumatic perinatal experiences and posttraumatic stress symptoms in midwives: prevalence and association with burnout. *Int J Nurs Stud* [Internet]. 2015;52(2):578–87. Available from: http://dx.doi.org/10.1016/j.ijnurstu.2014.11.006

2. Slade P, Sheen K, Collinge S, Butters J, Spiby H. A programme for the prevention of post-traumatic stress disorder in midwifery (POPPY): indications of effectiveness from a feasibility study. *Eur J Psychotraumatol* [Internet]. 2018;9(1):1518069. Available from: http://dx.doi.org/10.1080/20008198.2018.1518069

3. Leinweber J, Creedy DK, Rowe H, Gamble J. Responses to birth trauma and prevalence of posttraumatic stress among Australian midwives. *Women Birth* [Internet]. 2017;30(1):40–5. Available from: http://dx.doi.org/10.1016/j.wombi.2016.06.006

4. Patterson J, Hollins Martin CJ, Karatzias T. Disempowered midwives and traumatised women: Exploring the parallel processes of care provider interaction that contribute to women developing Post Traumatic Stress Disorder (PTSD) post childbirth. *Midwifery* [Internet]. 2019;76:21–35. Available from: http://dx.doi.org/10.1016/j.midw.2019.05.010

5. Sheen K, Spiby H, Slade P. Exposure to traumatic perinatal experiences and posttraumatic stress symptoms in midwives: prevalence and association with burnout. *Int J Nurs Stud* [Internet]. 2015;52(2):578–87. Available from: http://dx.doi.org/10.1016/j.ijnurstu.2014.11.006

6. Leinweber J, Creedy DK, Rowe H, Gamble J. Responses to birth trauma and prevalence of posttraumatic stress among Australian midwives. *Women Birth* [Internet]. 2017;30(1):40–5. Available from: http://dx.doi.org/10.1016/j.wombi.2016.06.006

7. Cankaya S, Erkal Aksoy Y, Dereli Yılmaz S. Midwives' experiences of witnessing traumatic hospital birth events: A qualitative study. *J Eval Clin Pract* [Internet]. 2021;27(4):847–57. Available from: http://dx.doi.org/10.1111/jep.13487

8. Uddin N, Ayers S, Khine R, Webb R. The perceived impact of birth trauma witnessed by maternity health professionals: A systematic review. *Midwifery* [Internet]. 2022;114(103460):103460. Available from: http://dx.doi.org/10.1016/j.midw.2022.103460

9. Campling P. Reforming the culture of healthcare: the case for intelligent kindness. *BJPsych Bull* [Internet]. 2015;39(1):1–5: p.1. Available from: http://dx.doi.org/10.1192/pb.bp.114.047449

10. Slade P, Balling K, Sheen K, Goodfellow L, Rymer J, Spiby H, et al. Work-related post-traumatic stress symptoms in obstetricians and gynaecologists: findings from INDIGO, a mixed-methods study with a cross-sectional survey and in-depth interviews. *BJOG* [Internet]. 2020;127(5):600–8. Available from: http://

dx.doi.org/10.1111/1471-0528.16076

11. Cankaya S, Erkal Aksoy Y, Dereli Yılmaz S. Midwives' experiences of witnessing traumatic hospital birth events: A qualitative study. *J Eval Clin Pract* [Internet]. 2021;27(4):847–57. Available from: http://dx.doi.org/10.1111/jep.13487

12. Rice H, Warland J. Bearing witness: midwives experiences of witnessing traumatic birth. *Midwifery* [Internet]. 2013;29(9):1056–63. Available from: http://dx.doi.org/10.1016/j.midw.2012.12.003

13. Sheen K, Spiby H, Slade P. What are the characteristics of perinatal events perceived to be traumatic by midwives? *Midwifery* [Internet]. 2016;40:55–61. Available from: http://dx.doi.org/10.1016/j.midw.2016.06.007

14. Sheen K, Spiby H, Slade P. The experience and impact of traumatic perinatal event experiences in midwives: A qualitative investigation. *Int J Nurs Stud* [Internet]. 2016;53:61–72. Available from: http://dx.doi.org/10.1016/j.ijnurstu.2015.10.003

15. Sheen K, Spiby H, Slade P. Exposure to traumatic perinatal experiences and posttraumatic stress symptoms in midwives: prevalence and association with burnout. *Int J Nurs Stud* [Internet]. 2015;52(2):578–87. Available from: http://dx.doi.org/10.1016/j.ijnurstu.2014.11.006

16. Garratt L. *Survivors of Childhood Sexual Abuse and Midwifery Practice: CSA, Birth and Powerlessness.* London, England: Routledge; 2011: p124

17. Garratt L. *Survivors of Childhood Sexual Abuse and Midwifery Practice: CSA, Birth and Powerlessness.* London, England: Routledge; 2011.

18. McDaniel LR, Morris C. The second victim phenomenon: How are midwives affected? *J Midwifery Womens Health* [Internet]. 2020;65(4):503–11. Available from: http://dx.doi.org/10.1111/jmwh.13092

19. Smith J. *Nurturing Maternity Staff: How to tackle trauma, stress and burnout to create a positive working culture in the NHS.* London, England: Pinter & Martin; 2022.

20. Levine P. *In an Unspoken Voice: How the Body Releases Trauma and Restores Goodness.* Berkeley. North Atlantic Books; 2010.

21. Levine P. *In an Unspoken Voice: How the Body Releases Trauma and Restores Goodness.* Berkeley. North Atlantic Books; 2010.

22. Acosta J, Prager JS. *The worst is over: verbal first aid to calm, relieve pain, promote healing and save lives* London. CreateSpace Independent Publishing Platform; 2014.

23. Levine P. *In an Unspoken Voice: How the Body Releases Trauma and Restores Goodness.* Berkeley. North Atlantic Books; 2010.

24. Van Der Kolk B. *The Body Keeps the Score: Mind Brain and Body in the Transformation of Trauma.* London: Penguin; 2015.

25. Kay A. *This is Going to Hurt.* Episode 2. BBC productions; 2022.

26. Van Der Kolk B. *The Body Keeps the Score: Mind Brain and Body in the Transformation of Trauma.* London: Penguin; 2015: p. 52

27. Van Der Kolk B. *The Body Keeps the Score: Mind Brain and Body in the Transformation of Trauma.* London: Penguin; 2015.

28. Slade P. Spiby H. Together we can care for each other. Online RCM conference; 2021, Oct 5.

29. Cankaya S, Erkal Aksoy Y, Dereli Yılmaz S. Midwives' experiences of witnessing traumatic hospital birth events: A qualitative study. *J Eval Clin Pract* [Internet]. 2021;27(4):847–57. Available from: http://dx.doi.org/10.1111/jep.13487

30. Weeks A. Post-traumatic stress disorder – part of our normal working life? 2021; Available from: https://www.rcog.org.uk/news/post-traumatic-stress-disorder-part-of-our-normal-working-life/

31. Slade P, Sheen K, Collinge S, Butters J, Spiby H. A programme for the prevention of post-traumatic stress disorder in midwifery (POPPY): indications of effectiveness from a feasibility study. *Eur J Psychotraumatol* [Internet]. 2018;9(1):1518069. Available from: http://dx.doi.org/10.1080/200081 98.2018.1518069

32. Read J. Personal communication; 2022

33. Brown B. *Daring Greatly: How the Courage to Be Vulnerable Transforms the Way We Live, Love, Parent, and Lead*. London: Penguin Life; 2015

34. Beck CT, Eaton CM, Gable RK. Vicarious posttraumatic growth in labor and delivery nurses. *J Obstet Gynecol Neonatal Nurs* [Internet]. 2016;45(6):801–12. Available from: http://dx.doi.org/10.1016/j.jogn.2016.07.008

35. Beck CT, Rivera J, Gable RK. A mixed-methods study of vicarious posttraumatic growth in certified nurse-midwives. *J Midwifery Womens Health* [Internet]. 2017;62(1):80–7. Available from: http://dx.doi.org/10.1111/jmwh.12523

36. Minooee S, Cummins A, Sims DJ, Foureur M, Travaglia J. Scoping review of the impact of birth trauma on clinical decisions of midwives. *J Eval Clin Pract* [Internet]. 2020;26(4):1270–9. Available from: http://dx.doi.org/10.1111/jep.13335

37. Tedeschi RG, Calhoun LG. The Posttraumatic Growth Inventory: measuring the positive legacy of trauma. *J Trauma Stress* [Internet]. 1996;9(3):455–71. Available from: http://dx.doi.org/10.1007/bf02103658

38. Patterson J, Hollins Martin CJ, Karatzias T. Disempowered midwives and traumatised women: Exploring the parallel processes of care provider interaction that contribute to women developing Post Traumatic Stress Disorder (PTSD) post childbirth. *Midwifery* [Internet]. 2019;76:21–35. Available from: http://dx.doi.org/10.1016/j.midw.2019.05.010

39. Minooee S, Cummins A, Sims DJ, Foureur M, Travaglia J. Scoping review of the impact of birth trauma on clinical decisions of midwives. *J Eval Clin Pract* [Internet]. 2020;26(4):1270–9. Available from: http://dx.doi.org/10.1111/jep.13335

40. Toohill J, Fenwick J, Sidebotham M, Gamble J, Creedy DK. Trauma and fear in Australian midwives. *Women Birth* [Internet]. 2019;32(1):64–71. Available from: http://dx.doi.org/10.1016/j.wombi.2018.04.003

41. Elmir R, Pangas J, Dahlen H, Schmied V. A meta-ethnographic synthesis of midwives and nurses experiences of adverse labour and birth events. *J Clin Nurs* [Internet]. 2017;26(23–24):4184–200. Available from: http://dx.doi.org/10.1111/jocn.13965

42. Birthrights report Systemic Racism, Not Broken Bodies: An inquiry into racial injustice and human rights in UK maternity care. 2022. Available from: https://www.birthrights.org.uk/wp-content/uploads/2022/05/Birthrights-inquiry-systemic-racism_exec-summary_May-22-web.pdf

43. Birthrights report Systemic Racism, Not Broken Bodies: An inquiry into racial injustice and human rights in UK maternity care. 2022. Available from: https://www.birthrights.org.uk/wp-content/uploads/2022/05/Birthrights-inquiry-systemic-racism_exec-summary_May-22-web.pdf

44. Birthrights report Systemic Racism, Not Broken Bodies: An inquiry into racial injustice and human rights in UK maternity care. 2022. Available from: https://www.birthrights.org.uk/wp-content/uploads/2022/05/Birthrights-inquiry-systemic-racism_exec-summary_May-22-web.pdf

45. Geronimus AT. The weathering hypothesis and the health of African-American women and infants: evidence and speculations. *Ethn Dis*. 1992 Summer;2(3):207–21.

46. Knight M, Bunch K, Patel R, Shakespeare J, Kotnis R, Kenyon S, Kurinczuk JJ (Eds.) on behalf of MBRRACE-UK. Saving Lives, Improving Mothers' Care Core Report - Lessons learned to inform maternity care from the UK and Ireland Confidential Enquiries into Maternal Deaths and Morbidity 2018-20. Oxford: National Perinatal Epidemiology Unit, University of Oxford 2022 [Internet]. www.npeu.ox.ac.uk. Available from: https://www.npeu.ox.ac.uk/assets/downloads/mbrrace-uk/reports/maternal-report-2022/MBRRACE-UK_Maternal_MAIN_Report_2022_v10.pdf

47. Draper ES, Gallimore ID, Smith LK, Matthews RJ, Fenton AC, Kurinczuk JJ, Smith PW, Manktelow BN, on behalf of the MBRRACE-UK Collaboration. MBRRACE-UK Perinatal Mortality Surveillance Report, UK Perinatal Deaths for Births from January to December 2020. Leicester: The Infant Mortality and Morbidity Studies, Department of Health Sciences, University of Leicester. 2022 [Internet]. Available from: https://www.npeu.ox.ac.uk/assets/downloads/mbrrace-uk/reports/perinatal-surveillance-report-2020/MBRRACE-UK_Perinatal_Surveillance_Report_2020.pdf

48. Knight M, Bunch K, Patel R, Shakespeare J, Kotnis R, Kenyon S, Kurinczuk JJ (Eds. ) on behalf of MBRRACE-UK. Saving Lives, Improving Mothers' Care Core Report - Lessons learned to inform maternity care from the UK and Ireland Confidential Enquiries into Maternal Deaths and Morbidity 2018-20. Oxford: National Perinatal Epidemiology Unit, University of Oxford 2022 [Internet]. www.npeu.ox.ac.uk. Available from: https://www.npeu.ox.ac.uk/assets/downloads/mbrrace-uk/reports/maternal-report-2022/MBRRACE-UK_Maternal_MAIN_Report_2022_v10.pdf

49. Birthrights report Systemic Racism, Not Broken Bodies: An inquiry into racial injustice and human rights in UK maternity care. 2022. Available from: https://www.birthrights.org.uk/wp-content/uploads/2022/05/Birthrights-inquiry-systemic-racism_exec-summary_May-22-web.pdf

50. RCOG. Racial Disparities in women's healthcare. RCOG position statement [Internet]. 2020 Mar. Available from: https://www.rcog.org.uk/media/qbtblxrx/racial-disparities-womens-healthcare-march-2020.pdf

51. Peter M, Wheeler R (with Awe T, Abe C. peer researchers) The Black Maternity Experiences Survey: A Nationwide Study of Black Women's Experiences of Maternity Services in the United Kingdom. Five X More [Internet]. 2022. Available from: https://static1.squarespace.com/static/5ee11f70fe99d54ddeb9ed4a/t/628a8756365828292ccb7712/1653245787911/The+Black+Maternity+Experience+Report.pdf

52. Dionne. Personal communication; 2021

53. NHS. NHS Workforce Race Equality Standard 2020 [Internet]. 2021. Available from: [online] https://www.england.nhs.uk/wp-content/uploads/2021/02/Workforce-Race-Equality-Standard-2020-report.pdf

54. RCM. BME midwives, disciplinary proceedings and the Workplace Race Equality Standard [Internet]. 2016. Available from: https://www.rcm.org.uk/media/5432/bme3.pdf

55. NHS Staff Survey 2021 [Internet]. 2022. Available from: [online] https://www.nhsstaffsurveys.com/results/

56. NHS. Turning the Tide report: The experiences of Black, Asian and Minority Ethnic NHS staff working in maternity services in England during and beyond the Covid-19 pandemic online [Internet]. 2020. Available from: https://www.northeastlondonhcp.nhs.uk/downloads/ourplans/Maternity/Turning%20the%20Tide%20Maternity%20Report%20-%202020.pdf

57. Alleyne A. *The Burden of Heritage: Hauntings of Generational Trauma on Black*

*Lives*. London: Karnac Books; 2022.

58. Health Education England. Capital Midwife: Anti-Racism Framework [Internet]. 2021. Available from: https://www.hee.nhs.uk/sites/default/files/documents/Antiracism%20Framework.xlsx, NMC and NHS England Combatting Racial Discrimination against Minority Ethnic Nurses, Midwives and Nursing Associates [Internet]. 2022. Available from https://www.england.nhs.uk/wp-content/uploads/2022/11/B1897-combatting-racial-discrimination-against-minority-ethnic-nurses-midwives-and-nursing-associates.pdf

59. Anwar N, Nazmeen B, Jones M, Okhamesan P. What We Need to Thrive: Experiences of Ethnically Marginalised Midwifery Professionals in the Workplace, Association of South Asian Midwives C.I.C (ASAM) & Society of African & Caribbean Midwives. 2021. Available from: https://static1.squarespace.com/static/5fc52bcaf7cf8c754046992e/t/6092d7853bb4505b999ac766/1620236167034/What+we+need+to+thrive_+ASAM+and+SoAC+report+2021+%283%29.pdf

60. Anwar N., Jones, M. What we need to thrive? [Internet]. Maternity & Midwifery Forum. 2021. Available from: https://www.maternityandmidwifery.co.uk/what-we-need-to-thrive/

61. Beal J. Microaggressions are as bad as overt hatred, NHS workers told. *Times* [Internet]. Available from: https://www.thetimes.co.uk/article/microaggressions-bad-overt-hatred-nhs-workers-told-bullying-58n39x6xd

62. Kinman G, Teoh K, Harriss A. *The Mental Health and Wellbeing of Nurses and Midwives in the United Kingdom*. London: The Society of Occupational Medicine. 2020. Available from: https://www.som.org.uk/sites/som.org.uk/files/The_Mental_Health_and_Wellbeing_of_Nurses_and_Midwives_in_the_United_Kingdom.pdf

63. Morrison T. Portland State, "Black Studies Center public dialogue. Pt. 2" May 30, 1975 [Internet]. 1975. Available from: https://soundcloud.com/portland-state-library/portland-state-black-studies-1?fbclid=IwAR1eh1xHKqm3zvG9Y4NMAMvWkFTle4-4uFhY4dahEFJQUrA2wCwjLVtwBNc

64. NHS. NHS Workforce Race Equality Standard 2020 [Internet]. 2021. Available from: [online] https://www.england.nhs.uk/wp-content/uploads/2021/02/Workforce-Race-Equality-Standard-2020-report.pdf

65. Ockenden D. Ockenden Report – Final Findings, Conclusions and Essential Actions from the Independent Review of Maternity Services at The Shrewsbury and Telford Hospital NHS Trust; March 2022. Available from: https://assets.publishing.service.gov.uk/government/uploads/system/uploads/attachment_data/file/1064302/Final-Ockenden-Report-web-accessible.pdf

66. Kirkup B. Reading the signals: Maternity and neonatal services in East Kent – the Report of the Independent Investigation; October 2022. Available from: https://assets.publishing.service.gov.uk/government/uploads/system/uploads/attachment_data/file/1111993/reading-the-signals-maternity-and-neonatal-services-in-east-kent_the-report-of-the-independent-investigation_web-accessible.pdf

67. Sciacchitano M, Goldstein MB, DiPlacido J. Stress, burnout and hardiness in R.T.s. *Radiol Technol*. 2001;72(4):321–8.

68. Mollart L, Skinner VM, Newing C, Foureur M. Factors that may influence midwives work-related stress and burnout. *Women Birth* [Internet]. 2013;26(1):26–32. Available from: http://dx.doi.org/10.1016/j.wombi.2011.08.002

69. Sheen K, Slade P, Spiby H. An integrative review of the impact of indirect trauma exposure in health professionals and potential issues of salience for midwives. *J Adv Nurs* [Internet]. 2014;70(4):729–43. Available from: http://

dx.doi.org/10.1111/jan.12274

70. Adriaenssens J, De Gucht V, Maes S. Determinants and prevalence of burnout in emergency nurses: A systematic review of 25 years of research. *Int J Nurs Stud* [Internet]. 2015;52(2):649–61. Available from: http://dx.doi.org/10.1016/j.ijnurstu.2014.11.004

71. Coldridge L, Davies S. "Am I too emotional for this job?" An exploration of student midwives' experiences of coping with traumatic events in the labour ward. *Midwifery* [Internet]. 2017;45:1–6: participant M6, p.4. Available from: http://dx.doi.org/10.1016/j.midw.2016.11.008

72. Power A, Mullan J. Vicarious birth trauma and post-traumatic stress disorder: Preparing and protecting student midwives. *Br J Midwifery* [Internet]. 2017;25(12):799–802. Available from: http://dx.doi.org/10.12968/bjom.2017.25.12.799

73. Davies S, Coldridge L. "No Man's Land": An exploration of the traumatic experiences of student midwives in practice. *Midwifery* [Internet]. 2015;31(9):858–64. Available from: http://dx.doi.org/10.1016/j.midw.2015.05.001

74. Davies S, Coldridge L. "No Man's Land": An exploration of the traumatic experiences of student midwives in practice. *Midwifery* [Internet]. 2015;31(9):858–64. Available from: http://dx.doi.org/10.1016/j.midw.2015.05.001

75. Coldridge L, Davies S. "Am I too emotional for this job?" An exploration of student midwives' experiences of coping with traumatic events in the labour ward. *Midwifery* [Internet]. 2017;45:1–6: p.4. Available from: http://dx.doi.org/10.1016/j.midw.2016.11.008

76. Spiby H, Sheen K, Collinge S, Maxwell C, Pollard K, Slade P. Preparing midwifery students for traumatic workplace events: Findings from the POPPY (programme for the prevention of posttraumatic stress disorder in midwifery) feasibility study. *Nurse Educ Today* [Internet]. 2018;71:226–32. Available from: http://dx.doi.org/10.1016/j.nedt.2018.09.024

77. Power A, Mullan J. Vicarious birth trauma and post-traumatic stress disorder: Preparing and protecting student midwives. *Br J Midwifery* [Internet]. 2017;25(12):799–802. Available from: http://dx.doi.org/10.12968/bjom.2017.25.12.799

78. Griffin J, Tyrrell I. *Human Givens: The New Approach to Emotional Health and Clear Thinking.* Chalvington: HG Publishing; 2013.

79. Hunter B, Warren L. Midwives' experiences of workplace resilience. *Midwifery* [Internet]. 2014;30(8):926–34. Available from: http://dx.doi.org/10.1016/j.midw.2014.03.010

80. Power A, Mullan J. Vicarious birth trauma and post-traumatic stress disorder: Preparing and protecting student midwives. *Br J Midwifery* [Internet]. 2017;25(12):799–802. Available from: http://dx.doi.org/10.12968/bjom.2017.25.12.799

81. Birthrights report Systemic Racism, Not Broken Bodies: An inquiry into racial injustice and human rights in UK maternity care. 2022. Available from: https://www.birthrights.org.uk/wp-content/uploads/2022/05/Birthrights-inquiry-systemic-racism_exec-summary_May-22-web.pdf

82. Davies S, Coldridge L. "No Man's Land": An exploration of the traumatic experiences of student midwives in practice. *Midwifery* [Internet]. 2015;31(9):858–64. Available from: http://dx.doi.org/10.1016/j.midw.2015.05.001

83. Coldridge L, Davies S. "Am I too emotional for this job?" An exploration of student midwives' experiences of coping with traumatic events in the labour ward. *Midwifery* [Internet]. 2017;45:1–6: p. 5. Available from: http://dx.doi.org/10.1016/j.midw.2016.11.008

**Chapter 9: Psychologically safe environments, compassionate leadership and incident handling**

1. HSIB. National report highlights impact and suggests improvements to reduce the risk of delays to critical interventions during birth [Internet]. HSIB. 2020. Available from: https://www.hsib.org.uk/news-and-events/national-report-highlights-impact-and-suggests-improvements-to-reduce-the-risk-of-delays-to-critical-interventions-during-birth/

2. Ockenden D. Ockenden Report – Final Findings, Conclusions and Essential Actions from the Independent Review of Maternity Services at The Shrewsbury and Telford Hospital NHS Trust; March 2022. Available from: https://assets.publishing.service.gov.uk/government/uploads/system/uploads/attachment_data/file/1064302/Final-Ockenden-Report-web-accessible.pdf

3. Smith J. *Nurturing Maternity Staff: How to tackle trauma, stress and burnout to create a positive working culture in the NHS*. London, England: Pinter & Martin; 2022: p.12

4. Kirkham, M. *Traumatised Midwives*. AIMS Journal 2007, Vol 19, No 1 Available from: https://www.aims.org.uk/journal/item/traumatised-midwives

5. Brown B. *Daring Greatly: How the Courage to Be Vulnerable Transforms the Way We Live, Love, Parent, and Lead*. London: Penguin Life; 2015

6. West MA. *Compassionate Leadership: Sustaining Wisdom, Humanity and Presence in Health and Social Care*. London: The Swirling Leaf Press; 2021

7. Edmondson AC. *The fearless organization: Creating psychological safety in the workplace for learning, innovation, and growth*. Nashville, TN: John Wiley & Sons; 2018.

8. Cardiff S, McCormack B, McCance T. Person-centred leadership: A relational approach to leadership derived through action research. *J Clin Nurs* [Internet]. 2018;27(15–16):3056–69. Available from: http://dx.doi.org/10.1111/jocn.14492

9. Ledger K. Person Centred and Compassionate Leadership. In: Smith J. *Nurturing Maternity Staff: How to tackle trauma, stress and burnout to create a positive working culture in the NHS*. London, England: Pinter & Martin; 2022.

10. O'Riordan S, O'Donoghue K, McNamara K. Interventions to improve wellbeing among obstetricians and midwives at Cork University Maternity Hospital. *Ir J Med Sci* [Internet]. 2020;189(2):701–9. Available from: http://dx.doi.org/10.1007/s11845-019-02098-1

11. Smith P. *The Emotional Labour of Nursing Revisited: Can Nurses Still Care?* London: Palgrave MacMillan; 2011.

12. Ledger K. Person Centred and Compassionate Leadership. In: Smith J. *Nurturing Maternity Staff: How to tackle trauma, stress and burnout to create a positive working culture in the NHS*. London, England: Pinter & Martin; 2022. pp50

13. Ledger K. Person Centred and Compassionate Leadership. In: Smith J. *Nurturing Maternity Staff: How to tackle trauma, stress and burnout to create a positive working culture in the NHS*. London, England: Pinter & Martin; 2022.

14. Brown B. *Atlas of the heart: Mapping meaningful connection and the language of human experience*. UK: London: Ebury Publishing; 2021. P. 122

15. Brown B. *Atlas of the heart: Mapping meaningful connection and the language of human experience*. UK: London: Ebury Publishing; 2021: p.123

16. Reed A. Personal communication; 2021.

17. Cummings GG, Tate K, Lee S, Wong CA, Paananen T, Micaroni SPM, et al. Leadership styles and outcome patterns for the nursing workforce and work environment: A systematic review. *Int J Nurs Stud* [Internet]. 2018;85:19–60. Available from: http://dx.doi.org/10.1016/j.ijnurstu.2018.04.016

18. Brown B. *Atlas of the heart: Mapping meaningful connection and the language of human experience*. UK: London: Ebury Publishing; 2021: p.172

19. Smith P. *The Emotional Labour of Nursing Revisited: Can Nurses Still Care?* London: Palgrave MacMillan; 2011.

20. Hill N. What leadership behaviours are needed to promote psychological safety in the workplace? Kingston University: London Unpublished MSc. thesis; 2021.

21. Smith J. *Nurturing Maternity Staff: How to tackle trauma, stress and burnout to create a positive working culture in the NHS*. London, England: Pinter & Martin; 2022: p.78

22. Feltman C. *The Thin Book of Trust: an essential primer for building trust at work* 2nd Edition Oregon. Thin Book Publishing; 2021: pp 9-11

23. Kitson-Reynolds E. The Lived Experience of Newly Qualified Midwives. [School of Health Sciences]: University of Southampton; 2010: p. 208

24. Cull J, Hunter B, Henley J, Fenwick J, Sidebotham M. "Overwhelmed and out of my depth": Responses from early career midwives in the United Kingdom to the Work, Health and Emotional Lives of Midwives study. *Women Birth* [Internet]. 2020;33(6):e549–57: MW 372 p.6. Available from: http://dx.doi.org/10.1016/j.wombi.2020.01.003

25. Feltman C. *The Thin Book of Trust: an essential primer for building trust at work* 2nd Edition Oregon. Thin Book Publishing; 2021.

26. Brown B. *Atlas of the heart: Mapping meaningful connection and the language of human experience*. UK: London: Ebury Publishing; 2021: p.50.

27. Smith J. *Nurturing Maternity Staff: How to tackle trauma, stress and burnout to create a positive working culture in the NHS*. London, England: Pinter & Martin; 2022.

28. Cummings GG, Tate K, Lee S, Wong CA, Paananen T, Micaroni SPM, et al. Leadership styles and outcome patterns for the nursing workforce and work environment: A systematic review. *Int J Nurs Stud* [Internet]. 2018;85:19–60. Available from: http://dx.doi.org/10.1016/j.ijnurstu.2018.04.016

29. Christoffersen L, Teigen J, Rønningstad C. Following-up midwives after adverse incidents: How front-line management practices help second victims. *Midwifery* [Internet]. 2020;85(102669): Interview 24 p. 4. Available from: http://dx.doi.org/10.1016/j.midw.2020.102669

30. Christoffersen L, Teigen J, Rønningstad C. Following-up midwives after adverse incidents: How front-line management practices help second victims. *Midwifery* [Internet]. 2020;85(102669): Interview 1 p. 4. Available from: http://dx.doi.org/10.1016/j.midw.2020.102669

31. Christoffersen L, Teigen J, Rønningstad C. Following-up midwives after adverse incidents: How front-line management practices help second victims. *Midwifery* [Internet]. 2020;85(102669): Interview 1 p. 4. Available from: http://dx.doi.org/10.1016/j.midw.2020.102669 Interview 1 pp4.)

32. Beck CT, Gable RK. A mixed methods study of secondary traumatic stress in labor and delivery nurses. *J Obstet Gynecol Neonatal Nurs* [Internet]. 2012;41(6):747–60: p752. Available from: http://dx.doi.org/10.1111/j.1552-6909.2012.01386.x

33. Christoffersen L, Teigen J, Rønningstad C. Following-up midwives after adverse incidents: How front-line management practices help second victims. *Midwifery* [Internet]. 2020;85(102669). Available from: http://dx.doi.org/10.1016/j.midw.2020.102669

34. Rose S, Bisson J, Churchill R, Wessely S. Psychological debriefing for preventing post traumatic stress disorder (PTSD). *Cochrane Database Syst Rev* [Internet]. 2002;(2):CD000560. Available from: http://dx.doi.

org/10.1002/14651858.CD000560 Kenardy J. The current status of psychological debriefing. *BMJ* [Internet]. 2000;321(7268):1032–3. Available from: http://dx.doi.org/10.1136/bmj.321.7268.1032

35.  Slade P. Spiby H. Together we can care for each other. Online RCM conference. Oct 5 2021.

36.  Christoffersen L, Teigen J, Rønningstad C. Following-up midwives after adverse incidents: How front-line management practices help second victims. *Midwifery* [Internet]. 2020;85(102669):102669. Available from: http://dx.doi.org/10.1016/j.midw.2020.102669

37.  Sheen K, Spiby H, Slade P. Exposure to traumatic perinatal experiences and posttraumatic stress symptoms in midwives: prevalence and association with burnout. *Int J Nurs Stud* [Internet]. 2015;52(2):578–87: Midwife 129: p69. Available from: http://dx.doi.org/10.1016/j.ijnurstu.2014.11.006

38.  Smith J. *Nurturing Maternity Staff: How to tackle trauma, stress and burnout to create a positive working culture in the NHS.* London, England: Pinter & Martin; 2022: p. 77

39.  Robertson JH, Thomson AM. A phenomenological study of the effects of clinical negligence litigation on midwives in England: the personal perspective. *Midwifery* [Internet]. 2014;30(3):e121-30. Available from: http://dx.doi.org/10.1016/j.midw.2013.12.003

40.  Robertson JH, Thomson AM. An exploration of the effects of clinical negligence litigation on the practice of midwives in England: A phenomenological study. *Midwifery* [Internet]. 2016;33:55–63. Available from: http://dx.doi.org/10.1016/j.midw.2015.10.005

41.  Hollins Martin CJ, Beaumont E, Norris G, Cullen G. Teaching Compassionate Mind Training to help midwives cope with traumatic clinical incidents. *Br J Midwifery* [Internet]. 2021;29(1):26–35. Available from: http://dx.doi.org/10.12968/bjom.2021.29.1.26

42.  All in the Mind,'Treating refugee mental health; Improving personal growth; Dream machine' (2022) BBC Radio 4, 10/5/22 [Online]. Available at https://www.bbc.co.uk/sounds/play/m0017451

43.  All in the Mind,'Treating refugee mental health; Improving personal growth; Dream machine' (2022) BBC Radio 4, 10/5/22 [Online]. Available at https://www.bbc.co.uk/sounds/play/m0017451

## Chapter 10: Resilience – really?

1.  Purser R. McMindfulness. Moral Matters Podcast Episode 22 with Dr. Wendy Dean and Dr. Simon Talbot; 2020.

2.  Purser R. McMindfulness: How Mindfulness Became the New Capitalist Spirituality. London: Repeater books; 2019.

3.  Purser R. McMindfulness. Moral Matters Podcast Episode 22 with Dr. Wendy Dean and Dr. Simon Talbot; 2020.

4.  Pratt S. What I Got So Wrong About Mindfulness and How It Might Transform Your Life with Dr Steve Pratt. You are Not a Frog Podcast Episode 116 with Dr. Rachel Morris; 2022

5.  Smith J. *Nurturing Maternity Staff: How to tackle trauma, stress and burnout to create a positive working culture in the NHS.* London, England: Pinter & Martin; 2022. p.17

6.  Hunter B, Warren L. Revisiting Resilience. *The Practising Midwife.* 2022;25:9–13. p.10.

7.  Crowther S, Hunter B, McAra-Couper J, Warren L, Gilkison A, Hunter M, Fielder A, Kirkham M. Sustainability and resilience in midwifery: A discussion

paper. *Midwifery* 2016 40:40-8. doi: 10.1016/j.midw.2016.06.005.

8.  Killian KD. Helping till it hurts? A multimethod study of compassion fatigue, burnout, and self-care in clinicians working with trauma survivors. *Traumatology.* [Internet]. 2008;14(2):32–44. Available from: http://dx.doi. org/10.1177/1534765608319083

9.  Croft, E. (2022) Factors affecting Resilience: the role of ACEs, a Coach-Athlete Relationship and Shift-and- Persist. Undergraduate dissertation, Newcastle University (unpublished)

10. Hunter B, Warren L. Revisiting Resilience. *The Practising Midwife.* 2022;25:9–13.

11. Hunter B, Warren L. Midwives' experiences of workplace resilience. *Midwifery* [Internet]. 2014;30(8):926–34. Available from: http://dx.doi.org/10.1016/j. midw.2014.03.010

12. Hunter B, Warren L. ****In: Byrom S, Downe S, editors. *The Roar Behind the Silence: why kindness, compassion and respect matter in maternity care.* London: Pinter & Martin; 2015. p. 111–5.

13. Grace. Personal communication; 2021

## Chapter 11: When midwives give birth

1.  Angelou M. *I know why the caged bird sings.* London, England: Virago Press; 2012.

2.  Charmer, L., Jefford, E., Jomeen, J. (2021) A scoping review of maternity care providers experience of primary trauma within their childbirthing journey, *Midwifery,* Volume 102, 103127. Available from: https://doi.org/10.1016/j. midw.2021.103127.

3.  Patterson J, Hollins Martin CJ, Karatzias T. Disempowered midwives and traumatised women: Exploring the parallel processes of care provider interaction that contribute to women developing Post Traumatic Stress Disorder (PTSD) post childbirth. *Midwifery* [Internet]. 2019;76:21–35. Available from: http://dx.doi.org/10.1016/j.midw.2019.05.010

4.  Toohill J, Fenwick J, Sidebotham M, Gamble J, Creedy DK. Trauma and fear in Australian midwives. *Women Birth* [Internet]. 2019;32(1):64–71. Available from: http://dx.doi.org/10.1016/j.wombi.2018.04.003

5.  Reed R, Sharman R, Inglis C. Women's descriptions of childbirth trauma relating to care provider actions and interactions. *BMC Pregnancy Childbirth* [Internet]. 2017;17(1):21. Available from: http://dx.doi.org/10.1186/s12884-016-1197-0

6.  Alcorn KL, O'Donovan A, Patrick JC, Creedy D, Devilly GJ. A prospective longitudinal study of the prevalence of post-traumatic stress disorder resulting from childbirth events. *Psychol Med* [Internet]. 2010;40(11):1849–59. Available from: http://dx.doi.org/10.1017/S0033291709992224

7.  Sheen K, Spiby H, Slade P. What are the characteristics of perinatal events perceived to be traumatic by midwives? *Midwifery* [Internet]. 2016;40:55–61. Available from: http://dx.doi.org/10.1016/j.midw.2016.06.007

8.  Toohill J, Fenwick J, Sidebotham M, Gamble J, Creedy DK. Trauma and fear in Australian midwives. *Women Birth* [Internet]. 2019;32(1):64–71. Available from: http://dx.doi.org/10.1016/j.wombi.2018.04.003

9.  Knight M, Bunch K, Patel R, Shakespeare J, Kotnis R, Kenyon S, Kurinczuk JJ (Eds.) on behalf of MBRRACE-UK. Saving Lives, Improving Mothers' Care Core Report - Lessons learned to inform maternity care from the UK and Ireland Confidential Enquiries into Maternal Deaths and Morbidity 2018-20. Oxford: National Perinatal Epidemiology Unit, University of Oxford 2022

[Internet]. www.npeu.ox.ac.uk. Available from: https://www.npeu.ox.ac.uk/assets/downloads/mbrrace-uk/reports/maternal-report-2022/MBRRACE-UK_Maternal_MAIN_Report_2022_v10.pdf

10. Draper ES, Gallimore ID, Smith LK, Matthews RJ, Fenton AC, Kurinczuk JJ, Smith PW, Manktelow BN, on behalf of the MBRRACE-UK Collaboration. MBRRACE-UK Perinatal Mortality Surveillance Report, UK Perinatal Deaths for Births from January to December 2020. Leicester: The Infant Mortality and Morbidity Studies, Department of Health Sciences, University of Leicester. 2022 [Internet]. Available from: https://www.npeu.ox.ac.uk/assets/downloads/mbrrace-uk/reports/perinatal-surveillance-report-2020/MBRRACE-UK_Perinatal_Surveillance_Report_2020.pdf

11. Peter M, Wheeler R (with Awe T, Abe C. peer researchers) The Black Maternity Experiences Survey: A Nationwide Study of Black Women's Experiences of Maternity Services in the United Kingdom. Five X More [Internet]. 2022. Available from: https://static1.squarespace.com/static/5ee11f70fe99d54ddeb9ed4a/t/628a8756365828292c cb7712/1653245787911/The+Black+Maternity+Experience+Report.pdf

**Part II**
**Introduction**

1. Brown B. *Atlas of the heart: Mapping meaningful connection and the language of human experience.* UK: London: Ebury Publishing; 2021: introduction ppxxix.

**Chapter 13: First principles: passion and purpose**

1. Lorde A. *Sister Outsider: Essays and Speeches.* Berkeley: The Crossing Press; 1984.
2. Brown B, *Dare to Lead: Brave Work. Tough Conversations. Whole Hearts.* London: Vermilion; 2018.
3. Leider R, Webber A. *Life Reimagined.* CA: Berrett-Koehler Publishers; 2013.
4. Bradshaw J, Brand Playgroup online course 2014
5. Kang Y, Strecher VJ, Kim E, Falk EB. Purpose in life and conflict-related neural responses during health decision-making. *Health Psychol* [Internet]. 2019;38(6):545–52. Available from: http://dx.doi.org/10.1037/hea0000729
6. Schippers M. IKIGAI: Reflection on life goals optimizes performance and happiness [Internet]. 2017. Available from: https://repub.eur.nl/pub/100484
7. Burrell T. A meaning to life: How a sense of purpose can keep you healthy. *New Scientist* [Internet]. 2017 Jan 25; Available from: https://www.newscientist.com/article/mg23331100-500-a-meaning-to-life-how-a-sense-of-purpose-can-keep-you-healthy/
8. Kemp N. Ikigai tribe. [Internet] 2022. Available from: https://ikigaitribe.com/ikigai/
9. Kemp N. Ikigai tribe podcast episode 5: Marc Winn On Merging Ikigai With The Venn Diagram of Purpose. Dec 29 2019. Available from: https://ikigaitribe.com/ikigai/podcast05/
10. Sinek S. *Start with Why: How Great Leaders Inspire Everyone To Take Action.* New York: Penguin; 2011
11. Chamine S. How we self-sabotage. [Internet] 2022. Available from: https://www.positiveintelligence.com/saboteurs/

**Chapter 14: In the whole of life**

1. Reed, A. Personal communication; 2021.

2.  Lorde A. *Sister Outsider: Essays and Speeches*. Berkeley: The Crossing Press; 1984.
3.  Mathieu F. Beyond Kale and Pedicures: Can we beat Burnout & Compassion Fatigue? [Internet] updated Aug 2021. Available from: https://www.tendacademy.ca/beyond-kale-and-pedicures/
4.  Brown B. *The gifts of imperfection: Let go of who you think you're supposed to be and embrace who you are*. Center City, PA: Hazelden Information & Educational Services; 2010: pp ix.
5.  Neff K. *Fierce Self-Compassion: How Women Can Harness Kindness to Speak Up, Claim Their Power*. London: Penguin Life; 2021
6.  Gilbert P. *The compassionate mind*. London, England: Constable; 2009.
7.  Kay A. *This is Going to Hurt*. BBC productions; 2022.
8.  Gilbert P. *The compassionate mind*. London, England: Constable; 2009.
9.  England P, Horowitz R. *Birthing from within*. London: Souvenir Press; 2007.
10. Cuddy A, Schultz SJ, Fosse NE. P-Curving a More Comprehensive Body of Research on Postural Feedback Reveals Clear Evidential Value for Power-Posing Effects: Reply to Simmons and Simonsohn *Psychological Science*. 2018;29:656–66. Available from: http://dx.doi.org/10.1177/0956797617746749
11. Cuddy A. *Presence: Bringing Your Boldest Self to Your Biggest Challenges*. London: Orion Pubishing Ltd; 2016.
12. Kabat-Zinn J. *Where You Go - There You Are - Mindfulness Meditation for Everyday Life*. Little Brown: London; 1994.
13. O'Donohue J. Poem 'For the Senses' from *Bless the Space Between Us: A Book of Blessings*. Harmony; 2008
14. Brown B. *Atlas of the heart: Mapping meaningful connection and the language of human experience*. UK: London: Ebury Publishing; 2021. p.214
15. Emmons RA. The psychology of gratitude: an introduction. In: Emmons RA, Mccullough ME, editors. Series in Affective science: *The Psychology of Gratitude*. Oxford: Oxford University Press; 2004 : pp.3-16
16. Emmons RA, Mishra A. Why gratitude enhances well-being. In: *Designing Positive Psychology*. Oxford University Press; 2011. p. 248–62
17. Korb A. *Upward Spiral: Using Neuroscience to Reverse the Course of Depression, One Small Change at a Time* London: New Harbinger. 2015
18. Hanson R, Shapiro S, Hutton-Thamm E, Hagerty MR, Sullivan KP. Learning to learn from positive experiences. *J Posit Psychol* [Internet]. 2021;1–12. Available from: http://dx.doi.org/10.1080/17439760.2021.2006759
19. Hanson R, Shapiro S, Hutton-Thamm E, Hagerty MR, Sullivan KP. Learning to learn from positive experiences. *J Posit Psychol* [Internet]. 2021;1–12. Available from: http://dx.doi.org/10.1080/17439760.2021.2006759
20. Seligman M, Steen T, Park N, Peterson C. Positive Psychology Progress: Empirical Validation of Interventions. *The American psychologist*. 2005; 60 (5). 410-21. Available from: https://doi.org/10.1037/0003-066X.60.5.410
21. Greater Good Science Center. The Science of Gratitude: White paper prepared for the John Templeton Foundation by the Greater Good Science Center at UC Berkeley. [Internet] 2018. Available from: https://www.templeton.org/wp-content/uploads/2018/05/Gratitude_whitepaper_fnl.pdf
22. 'Yours Sincerely' podcast with Jess Philips MP Available from: https://shows.acast.com/yours-sincerely-with-jess-phillips
23. Small K. Language Matters. Birth Small Talk blog [Internet]. 2022. Available from: https://birthsmalltalk.com/2022/05/11/language-matters/11/5/22
24. Ashworth E. Be Mindful of What You Say. AIMS Journal 2017 29 (2): 13-16. Available from: https://issuu.com/aims1/docs/aims29_282_29

25. Byrom S. Childbirth and the language we use: does it really matter?
    — [Internet] 2013. Available from: http://www.sheenabyrom.com/
    blog/2013/04/12/childbirth-and-the-language-we-use-does-it-really-matter,
    Ashworth E. Be Mindful of What You Say. AIMS Journal 2017 29 (2): 13-16.
    Available from: https://issuu.com/aims1/docs/aims29_282_29
26. Grace. Personal communication; 2021
27. Dweck C. *Mindset: Changing the way you think to fulfil your potential.* 6th
    edition. London: Robinson; 2017.
28. Kay A. *This is Going to Hurt.* BBC productions; 2022.
29. Mowbray C, Forshaw K, editors. *How to Rise: A Complete Resilience Manual.*
    London: Sheldon Press; 2021
30. Ellis A. Changing rational-emotive therapy (RET) to rational emotive behavior
    therapy (REBT). *J Ration Emot Cogn Behav Ther* [Internet]. 1995;13(2):85–9.
    Available from: http://dx.doi.org/10.1007/bf02354453
31. Brach T. Practice the RAIN meditation with Tara Brach [Internet]. Mindful.
    Mindful Communications & Such PBC; 2019 [cited 2022 May 1]. Available from:
    https://www.mindful.org/investigate-anxiety-with-tara-brachs-rain-practice/
    Brach, T. Blog - RAIN: A practice of radical compassion [Internet]. 2020.
    Available from: https://www.tarabrach.com/rain-practice-radical-compassion/

**Chapter 15: In the workplace**
1. Reed, A. personal communication; 2021.
2. Brown B. *Atlas of the heart: Mapping meaningful connection and the language of human experience.* UK: London: Ebury Publishing; 2021: p66
3. Otzelberger A. The Helper and the Helped: What Racism and Helping Others Have in Common [online] [Internet]. 2018. Available from: https://medium.com/the-good-jungle/the-helper-and-the-helped-what-racism-and-helping-others-have-in-common-and-what-we-can-do-14e52cfcb1d7
4. Byrom S. 'Midwives listen to your own and the mother's heart, as well as the baby's' Image. [Internet]. Sheena Byrom. 2018.
5. Cheek D. *Hypnosis: The Application of Ideomotor Techniques.* Boston, MA: Allyn & Bacon; 1995.
6. Fogg BJ. How you can use the power of celebration to make new habits stick [Internet]. ideas.ted.com. 2020. Available from: https://ideas.ted.com/how-you-can-use-the-power-of-celebration-to-make-new-habits-stick/
7. Fogg BJ. How you can use the power of celebration to make new habits stick [Internet]. ideas.ted.com. 2020. Available from: https://ideas.ted.com/how-you-can-use-the-power-of-celebration-to-make-new-habits-stick/
8. Hunter B, Warren L. Midwives' experiences of workplace resilience. *Midwifery* [Internet]. 2014;30(8):926–34: Midwife 3, p.929. Available from: http://dx.doi.org/10.1016/j.midw.2014.03.010
9. Mathieu F. *The compassion fatigue workbook: Creative tools for transforming compassion fatigue and vicarious traumatization.* New York: Routledge; 2012.
10. Siegel DJ. *The developing mind: How relationships and the brain interact to shape who we are.* New York: Guilford Press; 1999.
11. Ogden P, Minton K, Pain C. *Trauma and the body: A sensorimotor approach to psychotherapy.* New York; Norton; 2006.
12. Van Der Kolk B. *The Body Keeps the Score: Mind Brain and Body in the Transformation of Trauma.* London: Penguin; 2015.
13. Garratt L. *Survivors of Childhood Sexual Abuse and Midwifery Practice: CSA, Birth and Powerlessness.* London: Routledge; 2011.
14. Mathieu F. *The compassion fatigue workbook: Creative tools for transforming*

*compassion fatigue and vicarious traumatization.* New York: Routledge; 2012.

15. Mathieu F. *The compassion fatigue workbook: Creative tools for transforming compassion fatigue and vicarious traumatization.* New York: Routledge; 2012.

16. Brown B. *I thought it was just me (but it isn't): Making the journey from "what will people think?" to "I am enough."* New York: Gotham Books; 2007.

17. Brown B. Companion pdf to I thought it was just me (but it isn't): Making the Journey from "What Will People Think?" to "I Am Enough" [Internet]. Brené Brown. 2019. Available from: https://brenebrown.com/book/i-thought-it-was-just-me

## Chapter 16: Small change, big impact – how to engage in change

1. Grace. Personal communication; 2021

2. Johnstone C. Holding on to hope in the middle of a deluge of bad news about the world. 2012 Apr 13; Available from: https://www.theguardian.com/sustainable-business/resilience-hope-behaviour-bad-news

3. Dean W, Talbot SG. Physicians aren't 'burning out.' They're suffering from moral injury [Internet]. STAT. 2019. Available from: https://www.statnews.com/2018/07/26/physicians-not-burning-out-they-are-suffering-moral-injury/

4. Mestdagh E, Timmermans O, Fontein-Kuipers Y, Van Rompaey B. Proactive behaviour in midwifery practice: A qualitative overview based on midwives' perspectives. *Sex Reprod Healthc* [Internet]. 2019;20:87–92. Available from: http://dx.doi.org/10.1016/j.srhc.2019.04.002

5. Hunter B, Warren L. Midwives' experiences of workplace resilience. *Midwifery* [Internet]. 2014;30(8):926-34. Available from: http://dx.doi.org/10.1016/j.midw.2014.03.010

6. Cooperider D. The Process of Appreciative Inquiry. [Internet] Available from: https://www.davidcooperrider.com/ai-process/

7. Bridges W. *Transitions (40th anniversary): Making sense of life's changes.* Cambridge, MA: Da Capo Lifelong; 2019.

8. O'Donohue J. Poem 'For a Leader' from *Bless the Space Between Us: A Book of Blessings.* Harmony; 2008: p153

9. Kemp N. Ikigai tribe. [Internet] 2022. Available from: https://ikigaitribe.com/ikigai/

## Conclusion: going forward

1. Hunter B, Warren L. Midwives' experiences of workplace resilience. *Midwifery* [Internet]. 2014;30(8):926–34: Midwife 9, p .930. Available from: http://dx.doi.org/10.1016/j.midw.2014.03.010

2. Warren L. Personal communication; 2021.

3. Hunter B, Warren L. Midwives' experiences of workplace resilience. *Midwifery* [Internet]. 2014;30(8):926–34: Midwife 4 p.931. Available from: http://dx.doi.org/10.1016/j.midw.2014.03.010

4. Hunter B, Warren L. Midwives' experiences of workplace resilience. *Midwifery* [Internet]. 2014;30(8):926–34: Midwife 4 p.931.Available from: http://dx.doi.org/10.1016/j.midw.2014.03.010

5. Brown B. *Atlas of the heart: Mapping meaningful connection and the language of human experience.* UK: London: Ebury Publishing; 2021.

6. Brown B. *Atlas of the heart: Mapping meaningful connection and the language of human experience.* UK: London: Ebury Publishing; 2021: p.50

7. Gorman, A. The Hill We Climb: An Inaugural Poem for the Country. From *The Hill We Climb.* New York: Viking Press; 2021.

# INDEX

# Praise for *Flourish*

"Phenomenal, heartbreaking, soul-stirring... Reading Flourish evoked so much emotion in me – that 'oh my gosh, yes' conviction – stirred by the courage and compassion behind the words. Kate names the realities and lay them all out for the world to see and for us to finally let ourselves acknowledge. This holds power to trigger real change."
Katie, student midwife

"Kate has produced a book that acts as a guide, a reflective resource and a tool to amplify the voice of all midwives and what matters in everyday practice. Flourish is grounded in everyday reality, as well as theory and evidence."
Prof. Brendan McCormack, Head of School & Dean, Susan Wakil School of Nursing and Midwifery, The University of Sydney. Author of *Person-Centred Practice in Nursing and Health Care: Theory and Practice*

"This book is like a really good friend – empathetic and wise, coming alongside, full of helpful ideas expressed with clarity and kindness. Designed for midwives, but a wonderful resource for nurses and doctors too."
Liz Wiggins, Professor of Change and Leadership, Ashridge/ Hult Business School

"I love the way this book keeps things real. It does not shy away from the pain and contradiction of our healthcare system and yet offers each of us genuine hope; that against the odds we too might flourish."
Clare Cable, Chief Executive and Nurse Director, Queen's Nursing Institute Scotland

"Such a joy to read...like being under a warm blanket. Flourish is well researched, honest, convincing, expansive, and the tone is one of strength with ease and calm. The quotes and anecdotes are vivid and the illustrations are simply brilliant."
Pareena, student midwife

"An amazing book and immensely valuable!"
Clare Capito, National PMA lead, NHS England

*See also first page*